HEALING MEDICINE

A Physician Looks At the American Health Care Crisis

HEALING MEDICINE

A Physician Looks At the American Health Care Crisis

DR. SINE NOMINE, MD, FACS

HEALING MEDICINE

A Physician Looks At the American Health Care Crisis

Contents

A Note From The Author

When I made the decision to write a book about how to improve healthcare in America, I hesitated for some time. For years, actually. I realized that whenever any doctors try to improve a system, it is necessary to first point out flaws in that system. By extension, because people run these systems, we must often point to certain people and discuss what they are doing wrong.

My real fear was that readers would perceive my thoughts and ideas about improving the healthcare system as nothing more than whining by a doctor unhappy in her field. However, nothing could be further from the truth.

I love my job; I love being a surgeon. Having the opportunity to save the lives of breast cancer patients is a blessing. But, of course, just as in all professions, there are always a handful of people we encounter who make our jobs difficult at times. That is just a part of life.

But when these kinds of people become a weak link in an already flawed system, I do not think that we have any other choice if we want to improve the situation but to focus on that minority who compromise that system time and again. In the case of the healthcare system, these compromises can cost lives.

I am a lucky woman. A child of immigrants, I now operate a private surgical practice with my husband. Neither of us would have it any other way. We love our patients, the hospitals we work in, our co-workers in the office, and yes, even those pesky insurance companies. Most of the employees in these companies, and in all segments of the healthcare system, are competent, bright, compassionate people who do their damnedest every day to improve the lives of their patients.

However, "good" is never good enough when it comes to patient care. We must constantly seek to be as close to perfect as possible. It is in this spirit that I wrote this book. Perhaps it is a gripe-fest at times, but if my protesting and nit-picking can do anything to improve healthcare in America, then you could call me a happy doctor.

Disclaimer:
Names and identifying details have been changed to protect the privacy of individuals.

Introduction

When you take the oath as a doctor for the first time, you're committing to principles.

They're simple, but powerful. And you're making them part of who you are.

As a member of the medical profession,

I solemnly pledge to dedicate my life to the service of humanity; the health and well-being of my patient will be my first consideration;

I will respect the autonomy and dignity of my patient; I will maintain the utmost respect for human life;

I will not permit considerations of age, disease or disability, creed, ethnic origin, gender, nationality, political affiliation, race, sexual orientation, social standing, or any other factor to intervene between my duty and my patient;

I will respect the secrets that are confided in me, even after the patient has died;

I will practice my profession with conscience and dignity and in accordance with good medical practice;

I will foster the honor and noble traditions of the medical profession;

I will give to my teachers, colleagues, and students the respect and gratitude that is their due;

I will share my medical knowledge for the benefit of the patient and the advancement of healthcare;

I will attend to my own health, well-being, and abilities in order to provide care of the highest standard;

I will not use my medical knowledge to violate human rights and civil liberties, even under threat;

I make these promises solemnly, freely, and upon my honor.

The above words comprise our modern-day Hippocratic Oath. And its message has tremendous meaning to me. But our challenge as a nation is that our healthcare system—from the government regulations to billion-dollar healthcare systems to massive insurance companies to regional hospitals to the local surgeon and family doctor—seems to have lost sight of these values.

Too many of us healthcare professionals have become cogs in a wheel, invoices in a payment cycle, squares on an organizational chart, and unacceptable costs for a finance department.

And cogs, invoices, squares, and unacceptable costs don't heal a single patient. Personalized, dignified, high-quality care does.

I care about these things. I am proud to be a wife and a mother. And a surgeon.

From my earliest days as a little girl, I wanted to be a doctor. Growing up, I saw how my doctor cared for me, took care of my parents, knew me by name, spent time looking me in the eye, asked questions, and acted like I was the only person in the room. It was my dream job!

It inspired me to work hard, sacrifice time and devote my life to helping others.

I am blessed beyond measure and will always feel that way. But when it comes to medicine and serving those who need my care, I am concerned.

I'm not afraid. Nor dispirited. But I am anxious that too many in our healthcare systems are satisfied with mediocrity when excellence is possible. Or are focused on protecting the status quo when innovation and truly remarkable care is within reach.

I want us to do better, and I believe we must.

The status quo is unsustainable. It kills creativity. It causes us to lose vital talent every time a prospective medical student goes to Wall Street instead of into the halls of medicine. It tramples drive and enthusiasm, often with such ferociousness that more and more dedicated doctors are saying, "I'm out!" and taking an early retirement.

I've written this book to tell my story through experiences I've had over the years that identify challenges we face and to provide solutions that will make our system better.

You'll read about some of my frustrations—and trust me, we docs do get frustrated! But you'll also see my genuine passion for patients, who must be our priority.

Healthcare is funded by billion-dollar investments, but medicine is first a people business. Our humanity and concern for others can create amazing change. But if we become zombies in a faceless bureaucracy, our patients suffer.

Cancer patients, for instance, need help and innovation, not mountains of forms. Those with kidney failure shouldn't have to worry about a hospital's ability to staff a dialysis unit. Community healthcare options shouldn't be affected by arcane laws that are only there to protect big hospitals. And a patient's chance to fight for life shouldn't be halted because an insurance company's edicts say so.

If, like me, you want a better healthcare system, you need to understand the problems we face and the solutions that will make things better.

Our health and financial standing are interconnected. And the life we have one day may not be the same the next. It's up to all of us to do something to improve our society as the many brave doctors around the world have shown during the most difficult of times.

I'm passionate about this subject. It's my life and my purpose. I do, I've been told, have strong opinions. Also, I'm a sports mom, and you'll "hear" me in this book cheering, booing, and coaching. But fighting for the right things for my patients is just a part of who I am.

I hope you are just as motivated as I am to do your part to protect one of our most prized possessions: our health!

Lighting the "Match"— What Drives Me to Make Health Care Better

To understand my passion for making our healthcare system the best, you have to understand my journey to becoming a doctor and a wife and mother. It's a journey of hard work mixed with blood (literally), sweat, and most definitely some tears.

Let's start with "match day."

Little did I think about at that time how appropriate that term would turn out to be. Matches set fire to things!

Here's the way match day works in the medical field. When choosing your residency, fourth-year students pick their top choices of which residency they would like to attend. And the schools pick their top choices of students they want to attend. Then on match day, each student is "matched" with a school. And that school is where the medical student will perform his or her residency.

On my match day, I opened my envelope and saw a medical school far away and not one I had planned on. I actually panicked. Dreaming about it is different than do-ing it, and I was suddenly going far from home. I didn't let any of my med school classmates see my anxiety. Instead, I acted happy as I could be about the pick.

I rushed home to my apartment and immediately called my mother, nearly crying, and I said, "I can't go there. It's too far."

Without hesitation, Mom said, "Shut up. You picked it and that's where you're going!"

Mom never let me skate on my obligations, nor did she hesitate to express her opinions. I think I know where my opinionated streak comes from.

After three grueling years, I was a third-year surgical resident and getting ready to be on rotation for a month in the surgical intensive care unit. On this rotation, there were three residents: one from surgery, one from emergen-cy medicine, and one from anesthesia. And a medical stu-dent who rotated with us.

Before the rotation began, someone asked my chief res-ident if he could assign a medical student from another college to do this rotation with us.

I wasn't keen on the idea. I thought that one of "our" medical students, a personal friend of mine, should take precedence over an outside medical student, but the chief resident went ahead and signed up the interloping medical student.

Every morning at 5 a.m. the residents and medical students met at the x-ray board in the Surgical Intensive Care Unit (SICU) to start rounds. On the first day, I saw this six-foot, blond-haired guy at the board.

I walked up to him. "Are you the medical student rotating on SICU?"

He looked at me, kind of studying me, before flashing a crooked smile. "That's me."

"What do you expect to go into? Surgery, ER, or anesthesia?"

"Surgery."

"So you'll take a call with me," I said to him, then turned on my heels and walked off without another word. Frankly, I was still upset that my medical school friend was being kept in place of a student.

Despite my cold shoulder that day, I warmed up to him. So much so that I married him. And before long, two wonderful children would be on the way.

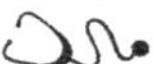

Although I'm only a bit older than my husband, I was three years ahead of him in medical school. I worked on staff at a medical center as an assistant professor of surgery while waiting for him to finish his residency.

When it was time to get a job as a practicing surgeon, three months pregnant with my first child, I started at a private practice. I lived in a studio-style hotel and paid weekly rent until my husband could finish his residency and join me.

My husband soon got a job but there were problems. During the first six months, he performed about twenty surgeries a week and earned nothing! Every month, his boss said, "Sorry. But your expenses were more than what you earned this month, so no paycheck." (These so-called expenses were the head surgeon's biopsy machine that only he used, biopsy supplies that only he used, all the cost of which were listed under my husband's expenses.)

That's when I learned that doctors don't follow the same labor laws as the rest of America, at least when it comes to other doctors. Just eight days before my second child was due, I was operating with a fellow employee from the private surgical practice where I was employed. We were doing a colon resection together. I had five breast cases to do later in the day at the community hospital across town.

But I started to feel what I thought were early muscle spasms.

I told the nurses in the OR that something was happening.

Finally, one of them said, "You're complaining about this every seven minutes!" Which we all then understood to mean I was going into labor.

Yes, I know how it sounds. The doctor was oblivious to the fact she was about to give birth! The nurses called my OB/GYN (all the way across town). They put the phone to my ear. I told my OB/GYN what was going on.

"Where are you at with the surgery?" he asked.

"The resection is done. My partner just has to close."

He said, "You need to get to my office ASAP!"

I called my husband and told him what was going on. He said something that only another doctor could understand. "I'm in the clinic, seeing patients. I can't leave to come get you."

Ugh.

The OR staff got me a wheelchair, and one of the orderlies wheeled me out. I drove twenty minutes to my OB's office, while having contractions every five minutes.

By the time I reached the office I was 10 cm dilated, which meant I needed to get to the hospital. I told the employees that my husband wouldn't be available to drive me, so they said they would call me an ambulance. They weren't letting the pregnant lady get behind the wheel.

I called my husband and gave him an update. Somehow, he managed to break away, driving me to the hospital just before the ambulance arrived. An hour later, we were parents. And not long after that blessed event, he kissed me and said, "I have to go do a gallbladder."

And I had to reschedule my five breast surgeries.

Within an hour of giving birth, the OR nurses I worked with arrived in my room with hands full of gifts from the surprise baby shower that was waiting for me which I obviously missed.

A few weeks later, my employer offered to hire my husband and bring him into our group. We were taking calls one out of every four nights (although I had been made to take calls every other night during the three weeks prior to delivery, and the three weeks after I returned to work following my second child's birth!).

The situation seemed more convenient in some ways, but my husband and I found that this employer wasn't doing much better about keeping their promises than his first employer. As frustration built, my husband gave our employers a ninety-day notice, which ticked them off. I'm not sure why, but they weren't happy.

My husband planned to start his own practice nearby. But it turned out we both had non-complete clauses in our contracts, which stated that upon our termination, we couldn't practice medicine within three counties until eighteen months passed.

So my husband decided to set up his practice just outside of the "forbidden radius," and one hour away from our home.

We decided to take a very much-needed vacation, although it still wasn't exactly a vacation. We used some of that "rest" to get my husband's contracts with all of the insurance companies rearranged. It was grim because we knew he wouldn't be able to bill anyone for the first three months of practice, as that's how long it took to get on the plans. But there was no choice.

Once our vacation ended, I performed four cases the first day back, one of them a bilateral mastectomy with a transverse rectus abdominal flap (TRAM) reconstruction on my breast cancer patient. It's a long operation, requiring a three-to-four-day hospital stay. After I finished the operations, I went back to my office to catch up on paperwork.

My boss called me into his office.

Out of the blue, he said, "You've been fired with cause, effective today."

I pressed to learn what the "cause" was, but he said nothing. I said, "I need to finish taking care of my patients, especially the one I operated on last who will be hospitalized for four days."

"But you're not working here anymore."

"But I need to take care of this breast cancer patient."

"You have a non-compete agreement. You can't see any of your patients, including the lady you have in the hospital. Another doctor will round on her."

I was stunned. "But I am her doctor. The patient doesn't even know that other doctor, and he is not a breast surgeon."

"Sorry. You're fired. You need to leave the office immediately." My boss's wife, the office manager, escorted me to my office, watched me pack up all my plaques, degrees, certificates, awards, and personal belongings, and put them into a big box. She escorted me out of the office in front of all the staff.

I felt like a criminal, but criminals at least know what they've been charged with. It was all very Kafkaesque.

So I drove home. I was out of a job, sitting in the living room, and hadn't received my ninety-day income that I was supposed to receive with termination. My husband hadn't been paid much of anything during his first gig, and he was just starting his own practice. He wouldn't have insurance plans to bill, and I had two toddlers.

I wanted to talk with my husband about what had happened. I knew it wasn't right, but I didn't know what to do about it. I didn't want my patients to think I had abandoned them, but I also didn't want to deal with my former employers suing me if I did see my patients.

I wasn't home an hour when two of my now-former staffers called. "When you resurface, we're coming with you!" they said. After we wrapped up the call, I hung up the phone and thought, if they believe in me, why shouldn't I? I decided to fight! I looked around for lawyers who would help me battle these income-crushing noncompete agreements and handle my wrongful termination.

As we would later learn, it turned out my employer was upset that my husband was leaving and expected me to do the same. They twisted enough arms to get three letters of complaint about me from community physicians.

One letter was from a woman I considered a friend who disagreed with a simple diagnosis I made. My diagnosis turned out to be correct, but my "friend" still disagreed enough to write a complaint.

The second complaint came about from a time when I was on call for Community Hospital, and a car accident patient came in. The ER physician called me and asked me to come see the patient.

Again, this doctor was angry with me. Or something. To this day, I can't figure out what I had done to upset him.

The third complaint was almost funny, even under the circumstances. Apparently, during a casual discussion with a referring family physician, I had called him "Bud."

How dare I! Seriously, that one was some kind of alternative universe thing. All of these complaints had been sent to the private surgeon (a man who was eventually kicked out of the hospital a few years later) who was my boss, not to the hospital committee.

So those three solicited complaints added up to the reason that I was, "fired with cause." These complaints, and a boss who was mad at me because my husband had left the practice, added up to some serious income issues for my family.

This put me in survival mode. The lawyers I spoke with said there was no way what I was accusing my boss of doing had actually happened, and that I would be better off going to practice far away because there was *no* chance I could win. But then I bumped into one of the CRNA's that I used to work with.

He said, "I heard what happened to you! It's pretty awful. I know a lawyer friend you should talk with. Here's his number. Call him as soon as possible. I told him all about your situation."

I called as soon as possible.

He told me, " You have a case here. I'll take it, and we will win."

It felt so good! For the first time, someone believed what I was saying and believed in me. We are best friends to this day.

Following my lawyer's advice, I collected dozens of letters of support from community doctors and my patients, stating that I was a vital part of the medical community and that my absence hurt patients.

In the meantime, my husband and I developed our own practice. I immediately hired the two employees who stood by my side. I got a large loan from the bank, rented space with a surgeon friend who used the office three days a week, and brought my patients' information from paperwork that my new employees had brought with them. Thankfully with all of those expenses and with people depending on us, patients soon followed! We operated differently, and our patients liked it. If we were out of network, we didn't charge patients the out of network fees. We treated them as *in* network and took whatever their insurance paid, even if it was zero. We even started taking ER calls at the local hospital, marching right into the teeth of the noncompete agreement. And that brought about, a few weeks later, an injunction letter from our former employer's law firm, which demanded that we meet ASAP at the courthouse. They wanted us shut down due to allegedly breaking the noncompete clause.

The showdown at the courthouse included my husband and me, three lawyers for him and two for us, and eight of my breast cancer patients.

The judge asked my former boss to take a stand. "Is it true that Dr. Nomine operated on breast cancer patients and you barred her from seeing them for follow-up? You didn't allow her to care for her patients?"

"Yes."

The judge looked shocked—at both the actions of our former employer and his smugness. I'm sure the judge expected this medical professional to put patient health before any personal vendetta. But here it was out in the open.

In response, one after another, my patients got up and told the judge that they love me and needed me. And I was the *only* surgeon within the three-county radius that had extra training in breast surgery, meaning I was the *only* breast surgeon specialist in the area. In other words, it would hurt the community to kick me out.

The result? We won and the injunction lost! This meant that we could stay open for one year until the final trial. Usually whoever wins the injunction wins the final case. Knowing this, my lawyer suggested we countersue our former employer for the ninety days' pay he owed us and for any bonuses we might have earned. But I was ready for closure. I offered to pay the lawyer $10,000 extra if he ended this mess within one week. He did. We got what we hoped for and moved on without a final trial.

I know our former employers stole money from us, but I just wanted my life back. I wanted to focus on my patients. We had spent a small fortune on legal fees, on top of the lost income. Not everything "turns out for the best," but this did. The women who came to work for us are still our friends. We have the honor of treating many patients every day and have the independence and lifestyle that we've worked for. It wasn't easy, but we love caring for our patients. It's what we do!

I didn't realize it at the time, but everything I just described shaped and sharpened my perspective as someone who saw the worst of our healthcare system but was committed to making it the best. When you're fired unfairly, you appreciate your job, but gain understanding of the unemployed. When sued, you gain perspective because you have "been there." But you also have expectations for doing things the right way—to reduce stress, avoid time wasters, and stop the foolishness and gameplaying that can harm patients.

But let me assure you, there are also some patients who make the physician's job a challenge.

The stories that follow will have you nodding with renewed understanding every time you hear that doctors are leaving medicine. Practicing medicine today can be both extraordinarily rewarding and immensely frustrating; you're going to read plenty of each in next few chapters.

Harper Hullaballoo and Mrs. Jackson Too!

One summer day I was finishing up office hours early. I'd worked a half day so my family and I could drive to see my daughter play basketball. I could write a book about the life of a basketball family, but that's for another time! This was her last summer in the tournament world, and I was excited to see the games. Sometimes a little too excited. I had one last meeting—with her school's high school athletic director— and then we would be on our way.

I hadn't eaten breakfast, so I was starving. I made my daily lunch: a fat-free turkey hotdog with ketchup, spicy mustard, sauerkraut on a honey-infused ballpark hot dog bun (175 calories!).

I tapped away on my computer with one hand, finishing up my patient chart notes for the day. It was moving along pretty well, the bite of hotdog tasted great, until my secretary, Nancy, hurried into my office and said, "Blue Cross is on the phone for you."

"Is it absolutely necessary? I need to wrap things up and get going."

Pamela frowned. "Yeah, I think so. It's about Mrs. Harper. She's griping about not getting a refund."

My first thought was, *no good deed goes unpunished.* But hold the phone: here's the backstory of Mrs. Harper. She was thirty-something, and a few months before flew to Florida to have a very expensive Brazilian butt lift in Miami. Then, back home, she had a fluid accumulation problem, which I'm sure was very painful. And of course, it worried her; she didn't need an infection, especially not there.

So, her primary care physician called our office and asked us to see Mrs. Harper that day. The doctor said the patient realized that since this was a complication of an elective surgery, it likely wouldn't be covered by insurance. But she needed to get it done. It would save her money to not have to fly down to Miami and get her plastic surgeon to fix it up.

We said okay, we'd do it. And then it all turned into a giant pain in my ass instead of hers.

When Mrs. Harper showed up, my assistant said, "We'll only charge you what Blue Cross would've paid us, not any extra. But, as a courtesy, we'll submit the claim to your insurance company and see if they pay. If they do, we'll just give you your money back."

"Great", Mrs. Harper said.

And why wouldn't she say great? She had everything to gain and nothing to lose. (Unlike, as it would turn out, me.) My husband saw Mrs. Harper and treated the fluid collection problem.

Mrs. Harper seemed thrilled. "Wow! You guys are wonderful. You saved me a bundle on a flight to Miami. I'm going to recommend you to everyone. I won't forget!"

She paid us $300. Cash. She probably spent that much on dinner on her trip to Florida. It wasn't going to make us rich, but she would soon be feeling better, and we had done our job.

All was well. Or was it?

A week later, Mrs. Harper's insurance company paid the claim! Not quite $300, but we weren't going to quibble. Then, a week after that, Mrs. Harper contacted us, saying she wanted her 300 bucks back.

With that news, Pamela and I looked up Mrs. Harper's account. Frankly, I was shocked that the insurance company had paid. I'm not sharing any earth-shattering news when I say that insurance companies aren't eager to pay any claim they get. I understand. Fraud is real. And that's from both sides, doctors and patients. Being careful is smart business.

But I was leery about this Mrs. Harper situation. Just like insurance companies, doctors in private practice have to watch our backs; it's a fine line between profit and loss.

I turned to Nancy. "Let's have the billing company double-check to make sure the claim won't be reviewed and turned into a 'billing error.'"

Here's why that's important. Nearly every week, we have about $500 taken away from us by insurance companies for monies paid to us "in error." For claims made going back as much as three years! We've even had to refund money back to the insurance company because the patient did not pay their insurance premiums.

Their letters state: "We paid you in error and it is the patient's responsibility to pay you this amount."

And then they take the money directly from our bank account. No waiting around for us to pay them. Boom! Gone! Oh, here's another thing: we have 30 to 60 days to file insurance claims, but insurance companies have three years to find their "mistakes" and take back our money.

Three years.

You can't make this stuff up.

We get prior authorization for a procedure, do our job for the patient, file a claim, and get paid. But then months or years later, the insurance company reviews a payment, calls it an error, and takes the money back from us, as though we're to blame. Not the customer. But they leave us all the expenses! And patients almost never pay us after their invoices says they owe nothing.

Guess what patients say when we try to bill them for work done months or years before?

"You're crazy!"

"This was two years ago? And you're just telling me about this now?"

"I'm sorry, you have the wrong number."

"You're a bunch of thieves!"

"Yeah, you can have the money. When you come over here and pry it from my hands."

So back to our Blue Cross phone call.

I picked up the phone and Tonya from Blue Cross said, "I understand you told Mrs. Harper that before you can give her a refund you need us to tell you that the claim was processed correctly and no refund would be forthcoming?"

"I do want to make sure you guys don't ask for a refund after we've given her a refund. Make sense?" I calmly replied.

She said, "I just want to document that you're doing this. This is fraud. You're keeping double pay."

The words knocked the wind out of me. I could feel my blood pressure rising. Somehow, our attempt to help others ended with a claims rep calling our actions "fraudulent," potentially getting me into legal trouble, and being banned from treating patients with Blue Cross coverage (which makes up about 60 percent of our patients).

I breathed deeply and said, "How dare you say this was fraudulent? Why did this claim get paid anyway? It's a complication from a cosmetic surgery."

"It was an emergency."

"No. It wasn't. She came to our office. She could've waited. She didn't want to fly down and see her plastic surgeon in Florida. So how could you at Blue Cross call it an emergency?"

Now a bit flustered herself, Tonya said, "I don't know, but it doesn't matter. The patient deserves her money back now. When will you be refunding?"

"But won't you guys take back the money when you review the case and see that it wasn't an emergency? Which will mean that we get paid nothing for services rendered?"

"It doesn't matter. The claim was paid. Give her money back."

"It can take up to a year for us get paid by an insurance company. So why can't the patient wait a few weeks until we make sure the claim was processed correctly?"

"I don't need to listen to this. I'm going to report you for not returning the patient's money immediately."

I struggled not to raise my voice and say what I was really thinking. "What is right away? Why would a patient need her money refunded immediately?"

Click. She hung up on me.

Of course, I was flustered and concerned. I ignored the charting and the staff meeting and I called my billing company. They were at lunch and wouldn't take my call.

I tried a few of my contacts at Blue Cross. Maybe they could help. The first one didn't answer so I left a message. The second one picked up. I explained the story.

She said, "I'm on vacation. I can't help you right now." I searched my mind for when she had been helpful before.

I said, "Can I just give you a number to call so you can look into it?"

She shouted, "I am on vacation!" Click. She hung up on me.

A few minutes later the other Blue Cross contact called back. She was nice. She got the patient's name and ID and said she would look into it and call me back shortly.

She did, but not with what I hoped to hear. "There's nothing I can do. You have to speak with somebody named Tonya. They won't even let me look at the case. Sorry."

I banged my head on the desk.

I called my billing company again and spoke to one of the reps.

He said, "I'll check to see if the claim was submitted as a nonemergency. I'll call you back."

I waited. I wasn't in a very productive mood, being seriously distracted and upset. I tapped my nails on the desk and waited until the billing company called a second time.

"We submitted the claim as a nonemergency."

Now I was seriously confused and monstrously frustrated. Why would the Blue Cross lady, the charming Tonya, tell me this claim had been submitted as an emergency and that's why it was paid?

The rep said, "I'll resubmit the claim and put in big letters that this was elective, not emergency. I'll call you when we hear something."

I wasn't done with the calls. I was supposed to be on the road by now, but I called Mrs. Harper's primary care physician. I told her the whole miserable story.

The GP said, "I don't understand. We did her a favor. She saved 600 bucks on flights to Miami and she's complaining about $300? I better be on my guard for her ripping me off, too."

By that point, it was mid-afternoon, and I was late for everything. I texted the athletic director, explaining why I was behind. I held a quick staff meeting and realized I hadn't had breakfast and never finished my gourmet hot dog lunch. Just to get it out of my mind, I told my staff to refund Mrs. Harper.

Later, I met with the athletic director, who asked me for a $5000 donation to the school's athletic department. In exchange, we'd get our surgical practice featured on a billboard in the high school gym.

I didn't need my surgical practice's name on the gym billboard. The ROI would be zero, but I do these things because that's what good doctors do—we give back. I was polite, but frustrated. I just had an ungrateful patient and a bully of an insurance company rep ruin my day, and now, in a high school I love—where my daughter is one of the best athletes—I was being asked for five grand! I took a deep breath and agreed but told him I would pay in installments.

I drove off to the tournament that day at least thinking I was done dealing with Harper-gate. But no.

A few weeks later, I got a notice from my bank that $25 had been withdrawn from my account. When I looked into it, I found the reason for the missing money. Mrs. Harper! She had called her credit card company disputing the $25 copay that she owed no matter what, even with Blue Cross paying for the office visit. So I called her and asked why she was disputing. She said, "You guys don't deserve a dime!"

In this instance, we lost money in time, effort, productivity (at least 10 hours of my time), and what Blue Cross took back from us due to "mistakenly" paying the claim.

So my dear reader, if you're wondering why doctor's billing practices are confusing and maddening, know that doctors are worried about their own Mrs. Harper in their practice and operate accordingly.

Everyone thinks a doctor's life is the greatest. Riches and respect. Caviar and country clubs.

Not exactly. It can be great, but the challenges are endless, responsibilities daunting, and the need for patience with a few unethical patients is unlimited.

If it were just Mrs. Harper, it would be one thing. But I can tell you that the virus of irresponsibility that is Mrs. Harper is contagious. Difficult patients are everywhere. Including Mrs. Jackson. Now she was really something. Let me explain.

Thursday morning. I had office hours until noon, after which I'd operate on one of my breast cancer patients.

At the front desk, Mrs. Jackson was checking in before her exam. My front desk receptionist came into my office and told me that Mrs. Jackson said she couldn't afford the $120 deductible on today's visit. Our policy is that copays, deductibles, and coinsurance fees are paid at the time of service. We ask patients to give us a credit card to put on file so that when the bill comes due, we can charge their card the agreed-upon amount until the account is fully paid. That's standard operating procedure.

"You still want to see her?"

As a caring doctor, I didn't want to turn her away. The exam took about 15 minutes, after which I said, "I need to see you next week for a follow-up."

My patient said, "Oh, next week? I can't. I'll be in Italy on vacation."

So she couldn't afford to pay me but could afford a two week Italian holiday. I guessed that the trip to Italy was going to cost a lot more than $120.

"So you can go on an Italian vacation but you can't pay your co-pay. You can't even give us a credit card to keep on file that will be declined until we push you further? Do you go through life paying for only what you want, not what you need? Is your health less important than European vacations? I guarantee that the airline you'll be flying on was paid up front, the hotel will be paid for, and any food you eat in Italy will be paid before you leave the restaurant. And if not, they'll lock you up! But if I, as a doctor, don't treat you right now, I'll feel guilty about it, and then I'll have to pay somebody else to collect what you owe us!"

(OK, I didn't actually say any of that, but it would have felt so good. I'm so glad we can't hear each other think!)

Instead, I told her that she could make an appointment up front for when she returned. Then when she walked out of the exam room, I called the front desk and told them to get a valid credit card number before we see her again.

I looked at the clock. If I didn't bolt out of the office like a felon being chased down by a police dog, I'd be late for surgery.

On the way out the door, I said to Mrs. Jackson, "Have a great vacation!"

Okay, I didn't really say that on the way out the door either. I wanted the fact she stiffed me to haunt her every sip of vino, but that wouldn't have been professional. I just hurried past my dear patient, biting my lip so I wouldn't say what I really thought. My lip really gets sore some days.

The irony of all of the Harper and Jackson stories is that the same patients who demand to be taken care of for free are the same patients that will be ready to "sue the doctor for millions" if anything (even if not the doctor's fault) goes wrong. It creates a dynamic in which health care is worth little if done correctly, but potentially worth millions to the unscrupulous patient and their lawyer, if ruled to be done "incorrectly." We are the offensive linemen of professions. No one notices our work until things go badly.

And despite no one noticing until bad things happen, doctors pay a heavy price to guard against that patient who seeks "jackpot justice" for even minor problems. Malpractice insurance is expensive! The average policy is $7500 for a primary care physician, while surgeons pay $30,000 to $50,000 per year to defend against being sued. That's after-tax money, which means a fixed cost of up to $200 per week for primary care physicians and up to $950 for some specialists. I realize few have sympathy for doctors earning low to mid six figure salaries, but think about that when you're considering why health care bills are so high. You're not just paying for your health care but are also paying for that of complete strangers.

I'm sorry. No one can work for free. No one does, for obvious reasons, and, as eager as most physicians are to provide excellent care, we all spent many years in college and med school and at internship, at great expense and self-sacrifice. We have rent to pay, mouths to feed, staff to employ, and insurance bills to pay. But some people just don't care and happily undermine the system. And when they do, they hurt all of us. Including you.

- In 2013, it was reported that there was at least $41 billion in unpaid medical bills that year alone.
- In 2018, it was estimated that collectively, Americans owe $81 billion in medical bills, and it's become one of the leading causes of bankruptcy in the country. One in six of us has a past-due medical bill, but thankfully many of us plan to pay it.

For those who truly can't pay their bills, I sympathize and understand. But for the Mrs. Harpers and Mrs. Jacksons of the world, I have migraines. How can they complain about a system that their actions compromise?

Mama-Daughter Drama

There's something memorable about mother-daughter days out—most are wonderful and then there's…a day with the McDonalds!

I was seeing a new patient for a possible left armpit mass. I had waited for the patient, Mrs. McDonald, to fill out her paperwork, which usually takes about 10 minutes, but this time took nearly 30.

I walked into the exam room, where she and her daughter were waiting. I looked at her past history. It said NONE. I looked at her medications, and it said NONE. I looked at her allergies and it said NONE.

Then I reviewed the referral sent over from the patient's general practitioner, which said the patient was taking numerous medications, including blood pressure meds and a blood thinner called Plavix. It said she had had surgery, a neck fusion, which had caused a metal plate to be inserted. This news made it almost certain that she couldn't have an MRI, information I'd like to know about in these types of situations.

I asked Mrs. McDonald, "Are you on any medications?"

"No."

"Plavix?"

"Yeah, I am on that." Sigh.

"Any allergies?" I asked.

She didn't answer directly, but looked over at her daughter, who sat silent.

"Well," I said, "What about penicillin and sulfa?"

"Oh those. Yes. I am allergic to them."

I wondered if I had lost my mind. I said, "It's very important that I know all of your allergies. Because if I don't know about your allergies, and then prescribe what you are allergic too, you can die. And then I'd be blamed because they'd say I should have known about your allergies."

Mrs. McDonald shrugged. I was hoping the word *die* would have some affect upon her, but no such luck.

"Alrighty then. Do you know why you have to take the Plavix?"

"Um, a blocked artery in my neck."

That would be a carotid artery stenosis.

"Why didn't you write that down for me?"

"I couldn't spell it."

I lowered my head and pinched the bridge of my nose in an effort to calm myself down and protect myself somehow from all this absurdity.

But I probably wasn't completely calm when I said, "Can you spell neck surgery? Or blood thinner? Or write down that you are allergic to some of the most common antibiotics? I mean, why would you write the word none in all of these sections?"

The patient shrugged again.

Her silent daughter, in her mid-30s I would guess, finally spoke up, apparently disgusted that I would ask for such private and esoteric information. "Look, give me the pen and I'll write them down."

"At this point," I said, "it's best that I get your mother's history and write everything down to make sure it all gets done."

I turned back to Mrs. McDonald. "Again, I can't stress how important this all is. I might have to do a biopsy on you, and not knowing you are on a powerful blood thinner, you could bleed excessively. Or if I would've ordered an MRI, not knowing you had a metal plate in your neck it could've been dangerous, even fatal."

Let those words sink in, because I'm not sure any of them actually sank in for the McDonalds. I obtained all the information I needed from them, examined her, and came up with a treatment plan. She'd have a study done and return in a month.

After they left, my front desk employees came into my office and said that the pair was livid when they left and said they'd never come in contact with a doctor as rude as me. They called me a "bitch," and would have the study done somewhere, but never return to my office.

"Her daughter knew all about this stuff, too," one of my staff said.

I asked, "What do you mean?"

"She's a nurse."

My jaw dropped. "She's a nurse?"

A really bad nurse. What's the old saying? What do you call the person who finishes last in their class, but passes? Nurse!

I couldn't believe what happened during this exam, but that the daughter was a nurse just stunned me. If anyone could understand the impact of leaving important information off of medical forms, you'd think a nurse would, right? Well, you would think.

Of course, had I given Mrs. McDonald a medication she was allergic to, or if there had been any other negative effects because of the lack of patient history, I bet her daughter would be the first in line to sue for negligence.

The daughter is the most disturbing part of this story. Nurses understand putting patients at risk, legal liability, the time shortage doctors have, the mutual respect that's necessary for proper health care to be administered, but she decided to ignore it all and act like she had never even seen a nurse before, much less was one.

If this is a medical professional, imagine what the amateurs do!

The good news is after they left, my next patient made my day. She told my staff, "Your doctor is the nicest, most amazing doctor I've ever seen in my life. I just love her!"

Those glimpses of appreciation keep me practicing medicine. For every bad patient, there are so many great ones.

Healing The Patient

I can talk all day about the need to make the health care system work better for patients. And you read patient stories that should make you shake your head in amazement, disgust, or confusion. But they're just symptoms of a bigger problem. We'll never have great health care until we cure what ails the health care consumer today—lack of savvy, information, or interest in caring about costs. And patients not realizing that not all medical options are equal.

If patients have no reason to shop smarter and think about quality, we won't improve anything. Patients need to have skin in the game to be invested in the outcome, and not just be bystanders!

There are five things patients can do to cure themselves of bad habits and lack of preparation that hurt them and the health care system.

1. Know When to Use-and Not Use-Emergency Rooms

The overuse of emergency rooms—the most expensive healthcare option for many healthcare services—is an epidemic. It starts with people not doing their homework and health care companies not doing enough to educate people about their options.

You can't imagine how many stories I've heard from colleagues and friends and the crazy stuff I've seen with my own eyes about people who show up at emergency rooms for sore throats and sniffles! Or less.

There was the parent who showed up at an ER frantic about a skin condition on their toddler that they were convinced was an emergency. Instead of a miracle being needed, a wipe with a tissue saved the day. It was the child's dried boogers all over their face, not the Plague!

And then add the patients who go to emergency rooms when they should call their doctor instead—or an urgent care clinic. And that's before we get to the serious challenge of too many emergency rooms being flooded by the mentally ill—a group who often need social workers or mental health professionals rather than ER care.

Also, many uninsured patients or patients with high deductible insurance plans use the ER so that they can get "free" care. Well, nothing is free. Someone is paying for it—You and me.

It's not rocket science, but consumers add billions to the cost of health care each year by choosing the wrong level of care for their problem. A 2010 report by the New England Health care Institute found that $38 billion was wasted in unnecessary trips to emergency rooms.

A 2019 report by health care consulting group Premier found that another $8.3 billion in health care costs were added by patients running to ERs for treatable, common, chronic conditions like asthma, pulmonary disease, diabetes, hypertension, heart failure, mental health, and substance abuse.

All of the above can normally be treated in non-ER conditions and make up about 60 percent of all ER visits annually. When you consider each ER visit, according to the Health Care Cost Institute, costs approximately $1917.00, you can see how much money can be saved if patients avoid ERs unnecessarily.

2. Get Regular Checkups and Preventive Care

I know. You don't like to go to the doctor. But if you don't go for preventive care and you don't take care of your body, you're a problem patient—and I want to cure you of that immediately. Doctor's orders!

According to the Centers for Disease Control (CDC), chronic diseases avoidable through preventive care make up 75 percent of U.S. health care spending and lower economic output by $260 billion per year. If everyone received the recommended clinical care, 100,000 lives every year could be saved. Reducing the percentage of people with high blood pressure by 5 percent would save the economy $25 billion, according to the Surgeon General's National Prevention Strategy.

For every HIV infection prevented, we can save $355,000 per patient. That's life-changing, lifesaving and about taking steps to prevent the preventable.

Prevention is worth a pound of cure and much more. Being smart with your body, being cautious, and getting the preventive health care you need will save you and everyone else thousands of dollars over the years! If you do all of these things, you'll cure a lot of patient-caused financial problems.

3. Get a Second Opinion—and Maybe a Third!

The U.S. health care system is one of the finest in the world and the leader in innovation, but humans make mistakes. Healing the health care system means reducing errors and patients have a role to play. That means when there's a serious problem, don't go with just one opinion. You wouldn't shop for a car without looking at your options and doing research, so don't skimp on asking questions regarding the best options to protect your health.

Misdiagnoses happen every day. David Eddy, MD, PhD, a health care economist and senior advisor for health policy and management for Kaiser Permanente, researched how frequently doctors disagree. He found the following:

+ Physicians looking at the same information will disagree with each other, and even themselves, from 10 to 50 percent of the time during every part of the medical care process.

+ Give a group of cardiologists a set of high-quality heart angiograms and they'll disagree about the diagnosis in nearly half of all cases. Individual doctors even disagree with their own decisions on two successive reads of the same angiograms almost onethird of the time!

+ Give surgeons a written description of a surgical problem, and half will recommend surgery. Of course, the other half will say no! Survey those surgeons two years later and 40 percent will disagree with their previous opinions!

Even in the most basic of treatment regiments, patients aren't guaranteed to get the care they deserve. According to research by Elizabeth McGlynn, PhD and Director of Rand's Center for Research on Quality in Health Care, most patients receive half the recommended services for treating common illnesses.

When all is said and done, it's up to you to fight for the best care. McGlynn found these disturbing statistics about the level of care patients receive:

- High-blood pressure patients receive approximately two-thirds of the recommended care.
- Nearly 75 percent of diabetes patients are not given essential blood sugar tests.
- One-third of heart attack patients receive aspirin, which is proven to reduce the risk of death and stroke.
- Under one-third of eligible patients are screened for colorectal cancer.

Some of that burden is on doctors but blame also falls directly on patients. Patients shouldn't diagnose themselves on the internet, but they need to be engaged and curious. Too much information—especially involving age-specific tests for cancers—is available online to be ignorant of basic facts. The best health care advocates for patients are the patients themselves.

If you're not getting the treatment you think you deserve, ask why!

4. Choose Your Doctor Wisely

Most people spend more time picking out a restaurant for dinner than they do deciding who will perform their surgery. I don't suggest you interview every person involved in your care, but you should understand that patients can learn a lot when they ask questions.

People shouldn't rely only on internet reviews, as they can be inaccurate and created by angry people who haven't paid their bills or upset about other things. But what I do urge is for patients to use their networks of friends, family, and contacts.

Happy, satisfied patients don't usually write reviews. But angry ones do. By nature, if we're mad about something, we're much more likely to tell the world! In my case, all of my negative reviews are patients who owe money, former disgruntled employees, and one person who wasn't a patient!

In that case where a non-patient reviewed me, I suspect it's a competitor who wants to lower my ratings.

Yes, it happens in restaurant reviews, on Amazon with book reviews and even happens with doctor reviews—competition might be online leaving bad ratings so they can look better.

Here are some things to know:

- A referral from your primary care doctor to a specialist doesn't necessarily mean the specialist is good. It can mean they have a business relationship. That's why going to a private practice rather than a hospital-owned doctor is better; hospital-owned doctors are required to send you to some specialists no matter how rude, expensive, or incompetent they are. Private practice doctors will send you to the specialists they believe are best for you. And private practice doctors get only about half the reimbursements that hospital owned doctors get due to contract negotiation leverage of the hospital's thousands of doctors vs the one or two doctors that lack of leverage in a private practice.

- Understand that every doctor's training is different, their interest in learning new techniques varies wildly, and they're never going to ever tell you they're using procedures from 20 years ago. You'll see this played out every day in a basic hernia surgery. Some surgeons only know how to do (or only have the equipment for) a procedure that involves a long incision, numerous stitches, and a long recovery time. Others are trained in modernized laparoscopic surgery that involves small incisions, no stitches, and a relatively short recovery time. have? And an even newer technique is robotic hernia surgery which involves an even smaller incision and quicker recovery time.

+ Talk to friends in health care about their opinions on doctors. Pros know who are the best and who don't measure up.

+ Understand insults/advice when you hear them. If you hear "you have the right to a second opinion" from a medical professional when you ask about a doctor's diagnosis, know that that this can be code for "go find help somewhere else!"

5. Be a Smart Health Care Shopper

Want to make a huge difference in improving the health care system? Start with caring about the price of the health care you get. While politicians continue to use health care as a club against each other, know that you can save money if you simply take ownership of your health care spending decisions.

Consumer driven health care plans aren't just in our future. For many, they are today's health care plans. Signed into law by President George W. Bush in 2003, Health Savings Accounts (HSAs), don't live on their own, as they're designed to be used with a high-deductible health insurance plan as a backstop against catastrophic health problems. HSAs can grow over time, as the contributions made into them by individuals and their employers can create health care money that can be used to pay health care bills in retirement! HSA usage has grown considerably over the years—some driven by consumers, but also from employers offering and incentivizing the use of HSA/high deductible health insurance plan pairings.

This is yet another way the insurance industry has duped us with a bait and switch. HSAs are designed to have the insurance company avoid paying for routine visits for non-catastrophic healthcare, which should make these visits affordable. Yet they are still expensive. I paid over $1500 a month for my HSA from BCBS with a $20,000 deductible. So, in effect, I paid my insurance company $18,000 a year in return for no health care services. The solution? The Government needs to limit what HSAs cost, just as they limit what I and other doctors receive for providing health care that saves lives.

In 2006, just a few years after their creation, approximately 5 percent of the workforce was covered by HSAs.

By 2010, that number had doubled to 10 percent of the workforce.

By 2016, 29 percent of employees were covered by an HSA, and that trend will keep growing in the future!

In financial terms, approximately $1.6 billion was deposited into HSAs in 2006 and by 2016, that number was

$31.5 billion. Imagine if this was all spent on health care. These are only the deductible amounts. The amounts the insurance company who you pay $100's if not $1000's to every month will not pay. How about if we all have HSA's? We all pay ourselves the full premiums and put the money in escrow so it can't be touched? When we go to the doctor, we pay from our HSAs. And anything left over? We, the patients, keep it. Not the generational wealthy insurance executive on his yacht wining and dining a congressman or senator with jurisdiction over health care laws.

How about we have health care money exchanged between doctors and patients directly? Without the insurance company who only works as a "roach motel"—money comes in, but rarely comes out.

What are the advantages for consumers with HSAs? While they're required to also have a high deductible health insurance plan along with it, HSA owners have major flexibility with their health care dollars. They can spend how and when they want. There's no "use it or lose it" concern that people have annually with Flexible Savings Accounts (FSAs), as the average 25-year-old who starts putting money into their HSA will see the unused money grow for decades until those senior years when health care costs skyrocket.

It gives people ownership over their future that reliance solely on Medicare never will.

To sum it up, how can you as a patient cure your part of health care? Get informed and be hands-on in decisions!

1. Find the right tools and use them correctly. Learn when to go to a doctor vs. an emergency room vs. an urgent care clinic. Know the difference and you'll save time and money.

2. Get the care you need when you need it. If you drag it out and don't get things done, it will cost you—and everyone else!

3. Do your research and don't hesitate to get other opinions and options.

4. Choose your doctors wisely.

5. Be a smart, empowered shopper, and find out options you might have (like self-pay polices) to make more of your health care decisions. My practice gives a 50 percent discount for our self-pay patients. Doctors aren't interested in gouging patients or becoming generationally wealthy. We just want to get paid for what we do and pay for our expenses.

Getting Sick of Health Insurance?

"Wait a second, another rejection from UHC? Another denial?" I said to my office manager. It was the third rejection in the last few weeks.

It felt like a mystery every bit as much as a major irritation. As my team and I looked at the information in front of us, in each instance in this cluster of payment denials we had contacted United Health care to see if a prior authorization was necessary for the patient's procedure. And in each, UHC had said no authorization was required.

But all of these claims were now denied because of no pre-authorization. We had called the number on the back of the card and confirmed that no authorization was necessary.

We subcontract out our billing process, so after some discussion, they contacted UHC to see what the problem was— and we then found out the issue. UHC was not the insurance company at all, according to their phone representatives.

We had been calling UHC, the company and phone number listed on the back of some patients' health care cards, but the actual health care company for these people was Alignment Health care. Alignment had put UHC's number on the back of their insurance cards, so that when a doctor's office like ours called for pre-authorization, the office would be told that pre-authorization, UHC would say it wasn't needed. Of course, it wasn't needed by UHC—they weren't the company insuring these patients!

Once we realized what was happening, we immediately called Alignment to get the pre-authorization. They rejected the claim. Every claim! And their excuse? We had not sought pre-authorization in a timely manner. But we had filed the claim—but were caught in a bait and switch filed-card con. There was no reason for this misinformation and confusion happening with patient insurance card information other than to do it on purpose. They even denied appendectomies for lack of prior authorization. Even if we had the correct information on the cards, there is no way to get authorization in the middle of the night for an emergency procedure like that.

It's all a ploy by some insurance companies to collect the premiums but never have to pay for the procedures that they claim patients are covered for.

And who else loses in this game? The doctors who end up providing the care, paying the expenses in advance, and then being denied payment.

It surprised me that the insurance company's actions were not prohibited by federal law. From pharmaceutical companies to doctors to hospitals, we're all under heavy regulation about false claims. And this one was a biggie.

But here we had intentional misleading of policyholders for the purpose of financial gain and we were left with no other path other than to complain amongst ourselves and apologize to the insurance company's own customers.

Outrageous!

As long as we let insurance companies get rich on the backs of doctors (who they don't hire, employ, pay for their education, or pay their expenses) and the patients who are the ones actually needing the care, nothing will matter. The bubble is so big and so much money is being made by businessmen and politicians that nothing will change, unless the insurance company clients, the doctor and hospitals stand up and say "no more!" We must insist there is no such thing as in-network and out-of-network. Either a doctor is qualified or not!

How the system would change if you, the patient, could go to whomever you like, control the health care premiums you've been paying to yourself, and you use those monies to pay for your health care. You would no longer pay tens of thousands of dollars over years to insurance companies, but pay only when you needed care! Imagine if you paid me (the doctor) $1000/month for 12 months and I never saw you as a patient. You would soon say enough and stop wasting your money.

And what if when you did need to see me, I told you, "That will be $300 because that's your deductible." You would laugh. Why do we let insurance companies do this? Why do we let insurance companies collect huge amounts of money (Blue Cross and Blue Shield, UHC, Cigna, and Aetna each made at least $1 Billion last year) that never help patients?

It's unbelievable that we've let this go on for so long.

But I don't want you to think that my concerns about insurance companies are all about money. Do they unfairly limit my ability to get paid for services I provide to my patients? Oh yes!

But my strongest feelings about them have to do with how they block or change the care I want to provide to those I treat. Don't mess with me about caring for my patients!

According to a poll by The Physicians Foundation in 2018, 38 percent of physicians said that regulations and insurance requirements create customer dissatisfaction and take them away from their intended purpose – to care for people.

Insurance companies have too much power in health care. They should be in the business of funding care, not determining what type of care patients get. But that's exactly what is happening. Health Insurance companies are not in the business to care for patients. They are in the business to make money. So don't be angry at them when they deny, deny, deny. That's just good business. We should, however, be angry at our government and the dishonest politicians who allow health insurance execs and politicians to gain generational wealth due to unethical business practices.

Our health care system is controlled and directed by "prior authorizations." When I started practicing medicine, I rarely had to get prior authorization for surgeries. Today, a bureaucrat in a cubicle is dictating what is available to you. This never-ending process takes up time for patients and doctors and can seriously compromise your quality of care.

Insurance companies also drive up our paperwork—or should I say computer work! They were instrumental in imposing the electronic mandates on doctors, which is a heavy burden for doctors and a cause of the breakdown in the doctor-patient relationship.

Doctors spend much of our time on EHRs in order to comply with meaningful use requirements. If we don't demonstrate that we're using a chart to improve patient care and communicate with insurers, we won't be reimbursed for appointments or receive government-set incentives. If we don't meet meaningful use requirements, we're penalized.

Some doctors working in a hospital setting say they've been asked to see one patient every 11 minutes, and The Atlantic reports that most doctors only spent 12 to 17 percent of their day with patients. The rest of the time is spent on paperwork, going over lab work, and interacting with staff.

So when you see your doctor typing away on their keyboard, understand that if we are not inputting the obscure details required, we may not get paid!

How else do health insurers make life difficult for patients, and by extension for doctors?

Insurance companies use prior authorization to avoid paying for certain treatments or medications. The process requires doctors to request approval from your insurance company before prescribing a specific medication or treatment. The treatment your doctor prescribes is often covered only if the insurance company approves it, based on their policies and without considering your clinical history.

While insurers say that prior authorization helps weed out medical errors and limits over prescription, studies show it leads to slower and less effective treatment and increased cost burdens on physicians. Knowing in advance that your doctor or nurse will need to fill out a prior authorization form for your insurer to cover your prescribed medicine or diagnostic tests helps set expectations. Expectations for a long wait, that is.

Those times when your prescription hasn't been filled and the delay seems unusual? It's normally because of preauthorizations, not because your doctor's office dropped the ball.

To cut costs, insurers use techniques like "step therapy" or "fail first" policies, which force patients to try cheaper drugs before the insurance company agrees to cover a more complex or expensive one. The insurer only covers medications prescribed by your doctor after the first drug fails to help.

This means insurance companies can require patients to take useless medications for months, which can put a patient's health at risk.

The extreme case is if a patient has not been helped by the first therapies, but then due to a change in employers or health insurers, has to restart the process, even though the first medicines may have been ineffective or caused a side effect or problem.

Another sneaky trick that the health insurance companies use is to exclude medications for their list of approved drugs. You see this happening more and more. Insurance companies are refusing to cover medications that they think are too expensive or claim are unnecessary. Patients have been denied treatments for serious illnesses, including diabetes and cancer in some cases. When this happens, follow the money. Why? Some drugs are excluded from lists because of financial incentives to keep them off. That means that someone somewhere has made a deal to help their company, but that's never a good deal for patients.

Also, insurers can force you to switch to a medication for non-medical reasons. They do this by eliminating coverage of the original medication, by co-pay coupons or forcing you to share a greater portion of the drugs cost.

In one study out of Tennessee, two-thirds of patients with chronic disease were forced by their insurer to switch medications. 95 percent said the switch made their symptoms worse and 68 percent said they had to try multiple new medications to find one that worked. That's not fair for anyone, especially those patients who rely on their doctor for the best advice. Instead, patients get the best advice from doctors that insurance companies are willing to approve.

These restrictions help you understand why some doctors—and some patients—are getting out of the business of dealing with insurance companies.

Some doctors have gone cash-only (check and credit card too), which means they completely avoid insurance companies. They often provide subscription services that allow people to get regular services for one low monthly price and some provide a menu of services with set pricing for both individuals and families.

What are the benefits of cash-only doctors? One is more one on one time with the doctor. It's an immediate win for patients who can finally have a conversation with their doctor again.

Another is price transparency. With cash-only, you know exactly what you're paying. And often, medications are often priced lower.

You can also get better care period because cash only doctors aren't held hostage to insurance company rules. They have flexibility to deliver personalized care that is best for the patient, not insurance companies.

Also, cash only doctors usually see fewer patients. And they can also be more flexible. In short, they do what they think is best for their patients.

There are some downsides. If you're already paying money for health insurance, paying more for a cash-only doctor may be painful. But some companies and families don't mind paying for the extra care. Also, the cash-only doctor care levels may not be appropriate for patients with very serious health problems. It's important to know what you're getting.

What haven't we talked about? The policies themselves—so many of them are too expensive, have too high a deductible, or don't cover what they should.

There are families—middle class, not upper income—who are paying $20,000 per year for their health care insurance. That is outrageous for many people who often use little to any of the benefits.

Then, you have deductibles that can be as high as $7000. Where does the average person find that kind of money? High deductible insurance policies weren't intended to be used by low-income people. They were theorized as good for people that use HSAs because they could draw from the accumulated funds, but not for the poor or those living paycheck to paycheck.

And some of the out-of-pocket costs don't end when people hit their deductible. In some plans currently, once people hit their deductibles, insurance companies begin to pay, but only partially. They share costs at that point, making affordability for many even less attainable.

Here's one more example of how money infects the system with the wrong priorities. One of my colleagues left medicine last month to work for a major health insurance company. He is going from caring for patients to denying claims and he will immediately get a $50,000 raise to work for the group that limits choices and makes life more difficult for his patients! Need I say more?

Staff Infections, Investigations and Disorderly Orderlies

Unfortunately, patients aren't the only problem, as sometimes we shoot ourselves in the foot. I've been fortunate to have many amazing employees throughout my time in medicine, but occasionally I have made some really dumb hiring mistakes. And when I did, my team and I have paid for it—figuratively and literally. And other times, I have had no say in who I was working with and I paid dearly too! Ah, the joy!

It was a Tuesday and I was getting a chart ready for a patient scheduled to come the next morning.

She had had an abnormal mammogram, on the right side, and the chart included her right-side mammogram, but not her bilateral screening. Generally, patients get a bilateral screening mammogram first. Then, if something suspicious is seen on one side, they go back and get more film done.

My rule is that everyone who comes into my office must have the most recent bilateral mammogram on the chart so I can confirm that the other breast has no issues.

So, I asked my staff, "Did this patient's primary care physician fax over the bilateral?"

They said "no."

I asked again later that day and was told that it still hadn't shown up.

The next morning, the day the patient was due for her appointment, I asked again.

Someone said, "They keep faxing over the wrong mammogram." That is, the right side, but not the bilateral.

This primary care physician was very good, and I was surprised I wasn't getting what I needed.

At that point, the patient showed up and was in the examining room. I walked in and told her, "We keep asking for the most recent bilateral mammogram, which we need, but they are only sending us over the right side. Please be patient and I'll look into it."

I stepped out of the exam room and asked my staff to call the patients' primary care physician again. He was out of the office.

So we got his nurse on the phone. I decided to take the call. "Hello, your patient is here in the examining room, but we've been waiting for days to get that bilateral mammogram. Can you send it now please?"

"Hang on," said the nurse. A moment later she came back on the phone. "We sent that at 8:44 a.m. We sent it days ago, but we sent it again."

I didn't want to argue. I put the nurse on hold a moment and grabbed the fax myself. It was a ninepage fax. On the first page I saw the right-side mammogram. Then, starting on page two, I saw the bilateral!

So all this time I had been asking for, searching for, and now the patient was waiting for, something that had been in our office for days. Sent just as it was supposed to be sent and when it was supposed to be sent.

I felt like a complete idiot. I got back on the phone and apologized profusely to the nurse.

Then I quietly—which wasn't easy for me after this mistake— asked my staff how we missed this mammogram so many times. It had cost us time and trouble, embarrassed us in the eyes of the other physician and his office, made us look foolish to our patient.

Someone said, "We're pretty busy here, you know." "And?" I said, awaiting a more thorough, not to mention reasonable, explanation for what had happened.

"I guess we only read the first page of the document." You know, because they were so busy.

They weren't too busy to keep requesting the document. They weren't too busy to talk to me about it. They were just too busy to look past page one!

As for me, they thought I had plenty of time to ask repeatedly where the report was, and call the referral physician's office to find out when and if the fax had been sent, and time to scroll through the fax to find the document we actually needed.

Often, to get away from things like billing drama, I like sorting through the mail. Silly, isn't it? I don't know why, but it distracts me because amidst the work that some mail involves, other things amuse or distract me. Coupons, thank you notes, and the occasional wrong address. Sure, it's mostly junk mail and bills, because, as Jerry Seinfeld once said, "That's what mail is."

One afternoon, I peeled open a letter from the IRS, addressed to my practice. That got my attention! I knew my taxes were in order but any letter from them is cause for concern.

It turned out that the notice had nothing to do with me or my practice. It concerned an employee of mine, let's call her Louise, and told me that I was obligated to garnish her wages for unpaid taxes. I could do it myself, filling out a ticket with the correct amount equal to 10 percent of her paycheck and mail it at, as they informed me, "my cost."

Maybe my payroll service could handle this. I called them. "Be glad to," said the payroll representative.

"Great!"

Then she told me about the fee. Of course, there was a fee. This was going to cost me one way or the other. Time. And money. It didn't seem to matter to the IRS that this was a tax my employee should have paid before I had even met her.

On to another letter. It was from my billing company, who sent me a list of patients with outstanding balances 90 days or more overdue. It added up to $200,000+ for the last few years.

So, after one insurance company denies half of what I had billed, another insurance company pays me a third of what I charge, another insurance company makes me bill the patient for deductible and coinsurance amounts actually owed to the insurance company, I still had over $200,000 due to me from patients. Ugh.

On to the rest of the mail. A malpractice insurance bill. That, I better damn well pay. Because lawyers, who claim to have only the best interests of patients in mind, only sue private doctors. Why, you ask? Because in most cases, government doctors can't be sued. Doctors who work for universities are immune to the tort system that takes money out of my pocket in malpractice insurance premiums, and then can take millions out of my pocket in a lawsuit ruling.

More and more, physicians spend less and less time with patients. More non-care work is piled onto our plate, generally by some faceless bureaucrats or corporate paper pushers, who don't care how illogical it is to assign busywork to people who are trained to save lives.

Like I said, sifting through the mail can relax me, but this wasn't one of those days!

Then there was the time a male, not mail, caused me grief with his delivery. Meet Abdul.

It was a Thursday afternoon, and I had finished my office hours at about noon. I met with my patient, who was about to undergo a double mastectomy with reconstruction after a breast cancer diagnosis, and then I headed for the surgical unit. I got myself ready for surgery and was at the sink scrubbing my hands. I spotted Abdul, the OR tech, and I said hello as he cleaned surgical equipment and restocked scrub masks and soap sponges. He was in his mid-50s, originally from a Persian country, and a Muslim. He knew I was an Arab-American Muslim. Despite the fact that I am a woman, and he probably had some difficulty treating women as equals, we had previously made small talk before surgery and he had always seemed friendly enough.

Some way or another we got to talking about names and what they mean.

I told him that my name means means thunder. He said to me, "My name means red."

Meaning no offense, I playfully said, "Well, actually, in Arabic, Abdul means jack A-S-S," spelling out the last three letters of the word jackass.

He looked upset.

Sympathetic, I smiled and said, "Hey, don't worry about it! Our names aren't our fault! They're something our families stick us with!"

We both laughed and I thought all was well. I thought wrong.

Later on, I started surgery, making an incision at the patient's chest wall. Suddenly, Abdul burst into the operating room, pushed aside the anesthesiologist, stuck his head over the drape that covered the patient's head, and shouted, "Don't ever disgrace my family again!"

Of course, everybody in the OR looked wide-eyed and shocked. I mean, we were in mid-surgery!

All I could manage to say to this crazy person was, "What are you talking about?"

At that point, I had no idea why he rushed into the operating room like a madman; my mind was on the surgery, not on a casual conversation. And that moment, the important thing was to keep my composure and operate as nonplussed and competently as humanly possible.

I put it out of my mind and focused on the task at hand: completing a successful operation.

After surgery, I went to the locker room, changed my clothes, and headed for the door. But in the hallway, a hospital administrative assistant said, "Doc, you're in trouble. You need to see the big boss right away." She was talking about our CEO.

I marched into his office and asked, "What have I done?"

"You upset Abdul today when you called him a jackass. He had to leave the hospital and couldn't finish his shift."

Abdul, who no doubt considered himself a strong Muslim man, had turned out to be quite the delicate flower if he couldn't even finish his shift because I had correctly translated the Arabic meaning of his name. And it wasn't like I made it up. I'm blunt, but I was not meaning to upset him.

"I did not call him a jackass. I told him what his name means in Arabic. I even spelled out the last three letters. We were joking and he didn't seem upset." I meant no disrespect and pride myself on the casual conversations I have with the staff every day.

"Well, he was."

"Did somebody also tell you he stormed into the OR, shouting and disrupting my procedure, and potentially putting my patient in danger? I finished my operation successfully, but his actions were inexcusable, and frankly, loony. What are you gonna do about that?"

Apparently, the answer was "nothing." The CEO said, "Your behavior was unacceptable. You're on thin ice now because you've harassed my employee."

"Are you telling me this was harassment? You're not serious. I harassed him? By telling him what his name means in English?"

"You need to apologize."

I knew the odds were stacked against me, so I took a minute to calm myself and accepted the fact I was in the Disney World of political correctness. I said "Fine. I never meant to offend the man. Please call him right now so I can apologize directly."

The CEO brightened, grabbed the phone, and called Abdul. "Abdul, the doctor is here in my office and wants to apologize to you." The CEO listened a moment, and then said, "Okay. Will do. Bye."

Then the CEO sat there, staring at me.

"Well?" I finally said.

"He said he can't speak with you right now because he's praying." Unbelievable.

"He's praying?"

"Apparently."

"Have you ever, in your history of this job, ever had an employee refuse to take a call because they were praying?"

The CEO shrugged lamely.

I said, "You're telling me that he had to storm into the OR, shouting like a madman and making a scene and endangering the patient's life, that he left work without completing a shift, and had to go home and pray because he was so devastated by the very definition of his own name? Then when the phone rings, he's not too busy praying to answer it, but he is too busy praying to speak with me and accept my apology? An apology that he shouldn't even need if he were not acting like a drama queen?"

The CEO sighed and sat back in his chair. "Here's what we'll do. I'll send you a letter reprimanding you for your abusive behavior. Make sure you do a lot of soul-searching before you write back to me and make sure it's an acceptable response."

First, it was harassment, now it was abusive behavior. By the next morning, I was certain I'd be accused of first-degree murder. In fact, the CEO had no idea what was really going on in Abdul's mind. But I did.

Abdul was a middle-aged Muslim from Iran. Women are second-class citizens in that country. Here I was, a Muslim Palestinian-American woman, apparently speaking disrespectfully to a superior being (a man). Yes, I could have chosen not to translate his name, considering. But I guarantee you, had I been the usual blonde traditional American woman, he would've just chalked it up to me being someone who didn't know any better. But I'm a Muslim-American female. He thought he was my superior, despite the fact that I was a surgeon and he was an OR tech. In his thinking, I should've known better than to joke with him.

In the hospital's letter to me, they accused me of discriminating against Abdul, harassment, and abusive behavior. I disagreed strongly with the last two but discrimination bordered on the surreal. How does a Muslim discriminate against a Muslim? I think he was just upset I didn't cover my head and kiss his feet.

And, unbelievably, Abdul received no reprimand for bursting into the OR! Few actions could be more potentially dire. Yet he wasn't even verbally corrected by hospital administrators about his actions.

At least one person in the hospital got it right eventually. The anesthesiologist came up to me weeks later and told me that he had read a great book on Islam, and he now understood that Abdul had talked down to me and treated me with little respect because I was a Muslim woman.

"He didn't see you as a surgeon. He saw you as inferior."

I appreciated those understanding words. But in the end, I became the bad guy in my superior's eyes and in my employee file. And Abdul? He was suddenly a loyal employee who had been harassed, abused, and discriminated against.

Can't make this stuff up, folks.

What occurred with Abdul is all too typical in the health care field, but it's problematic everywhere. Too many leaders base their decisions on what is the least embarrassing outcome rather than deciding what is the right outcome.

And I'm certain that the CEO smelled a potential lawsuit coming from Abdul and decided to lower the risk of that happening by forcing me to walk the plank.

With any personnel matter, there is usually a lawyer somewhere whispering to someone in power, "Make this problem go away!" And when CEOs follow those directions, they only create more Abduls who want their petty grievances catered to.

The medical field is held to a higher standard than most professional industries, and should be. Actions taken by health care workers can be matters of life and death. And though all of us are human and none of us perfect, we must do our best to maximize our knowledge, minimize potentially costly errors and provide the best care possible.

Nonetheless, health care has its slackers, and "suffers" from those who don't care enough about their job and about their patients.

Like every physician, I have examples to share. Lots and lots of examples, but I'll share just a few.

One day, I noticed that a patient coming in had faxed over her mammograms, except for the one that I needed to see most of all. The document downloaded into this patient's chart was 20 pages long, yet my staff said we still didn't have what I needed!

Front desk employees are supposed to make sure all referrals have the most recent mammograms sent over before an office visit. It's standard procedure.

So, I had to call the front desk and ask for the newest mammogram, which had been performed on August 22. The secretary proceeded to print out the same 20 pages — all the mammograms and ultrasounds that were in the chart and all the dates, except for the one I had asked for! Again!

And yes, I had just finished telling her that the 20 pages we already had were of no use to me, and that I needed the newest mammogram. A mammogram report is two to three pages long at most, so even if she didn't bother to take a look at the 20 pages she had just printed out, why would she believe that the 20 pages was a single mammogram report?

Also, another rule in our office is that all post-op patients must have the pathology reports in their chart prior to their office visit. Mind you, this is nothing special nor unique to my office. It's basic medical practice 101.

No-brainer, right? Wrong.

I was reviewing one of my post-op patient's charts, and noticed that the pathology report, which had been produced on March 8th, was not in the chart. Her post-op visit was going to be on March 14th, so there should have been plenty of time for us to get it back from the hospital.

Here we go again.

I asked my secretary to have the March report downloaded and printed out. She proceeded to add to the chart a pathology report from January. One that, of course, was already in the chart.

You might well ask why she didn't say to herself, "Wow! Why would the doc ask me to download and print out a report she already has?"

Or better yet, "Why am I printing out a pathology report three months old considering that this is the patient's first post-op visit?"

But no. She not only didn't log into the hospital website to download the report I needed, but printed out the old report and didn't even bother to read it.

Look, anyone assisting doctors with medications, needles, surgical tools, reports, should feel obligated to make sure that they have the right information or tools on hand before they give anything to the doctor. Because in some cases, it's the difference between life and death.

Every moment I spend trying to make up for someone else's laziness or carelessness is time I could spend treating a patient. And that frustrates me.

People reading this chapter may say "Pay more and you could find better workers." Well, that's hard to do when doctors have our income cut yearly because of federal rate cuts for surgical procedures. How can we pay more when we're earning less and costs are going up? When IBM increases employee wages, they pass it along to consumers through price increases.

Doctors can't do that because of federally set reimbursement rates. It's a zero-sum proposition for how much we earn unless we clone ourselves. We can't charge patients more because we renovated our office to make it more comfortable, gave our employees' raises, or we purchased a great, new $50,000.00 machine that patients will benefit from. It's sad that making life better for patients arguably makes life worse for doctors.

It was Wednesday morning and our busiest day in the office. Both doctors —my husband and I— were seeing patients all day.

About 10 a.m., I noticed one of my patient's electronic charts did not have her photo ID included. It still had that generic egg-shape face we've all gotten used to seeing.

Our rule is that all patients prior to being taken back to an examining room to be seen by the doctor, must have their driver's license ID scanned into the chart.

Up front, Jenna was training with Agatha. It was her second day being in front, and her eighth day on the job.

I approached her and nonchalantly said, "Agatha, this patient does not have a photo ID scanned into their chart."

She turned to me like I'd just insulted her parentage and said, "I didn't check that patient in!" Loudly.

"Aren't you training Jenna?"

"Of course."

"Then you know you're supposed to check all charts before the patients go back to the exam rooms."

This time, "loudly," became more of a shout: "I can't do everything, Doctor. I'm only one person!"

I'm not often speechless, but I was this time. You'd think I asked her to do the books, examine my patients, make lunch, change my oil, and solve the opioid crisis all in one fell swoop. But of course, all I asked was why she hadn't made sure that the patient's ID had been scanned into her chart.

My thoughts ran back in time to two great ladies I'd had at the front desk, who managed to do nearly everything themselves. If one wasn't around, the other picked up the slack!

During interviews before Agatha was hired, she assured me that she was a great multitasker and could handle anything that came her way. I realize that people may fib or exaggerate a bit during interviews, but come on, man. You had one job!

Jenna stepped up to take the blame. "Sorry, it's my fault." So, props to her.

I said, "Jenna, no worries. It's only your second day." But Agatha wasn't getting off the hook that easily.

I noticed that my patient had been listening and was rolling her eyes, letting me know what she thought of my crackerjack front desk person. Wanting to avoid any further escalation of an already ridiculous situation, I approached the patient myself.

"Can I get your ID?"

She smiled, glancing back and forth from me to Agatha. "I wasn't asked to do this when I checked in."

"I'm sorry. We're in training."

The patient smiled again and shook her head gently, as if saying, "My sympathies."

Then I asked another employee to make sure the patient's photo ID was scanned into her chart.

So, I got that handled. But the fun and games were just beginning.

Around 11 a.m., I noticed that Agatha had written on someone's chart that they owed 25 percent coinsurance of any services done. When that's the case, our rule is that an estimate gets printed out with the likely charges that will occur (I tell the staff what I think I will be doing to the patient prior to the appointment).

This way, the patient and I both have an estimate of what the patient will owe.

So, I approached Agatha again. *Bet this goes well.*

"Where's the estimate?"

Wildly insulted by my apparently outrageous inquiry, Agatha snapped, "She has secondary insurance, so she owes nothing."

Choking back my frustration, I said, "Agatha, if the secondary insurance has a deductible, then the patient will owe the deductible."

"She has secondary insurance, so she doesn't owe anything!" she said.

Mind you, we often have patients with secondary insurances who do owe their secondary deductibles, which make up a significant amount of our "unpaid accounts receivables." And the unpaid invoices skyrocket when patients are surprised by what they owe.

Once again, the patient could hear my assistant's loud protests. I wondered if she thought I was trying to rip her off. And of course, I wondered if she'd think of me in a negative light, because my staff was talking back to me. It's tough for a patient to respect the doctor if her own staff doesn't.

I tried to figure out what to do about Agatha, but for the moment, I simply wanted to avoid another scene. Yes, I was angry and embarrassed that I had hired an employee who not only did not do the job that she was hired for but showed me no respect in front of patients. It wasn't about her being right or wrong at this point; it was all about her attitude and big mouth.

I said, "I guess I'm just stupid." I wasn't, but I thought I'd just leave it there.

But we weren't done.

I saw the patient and had a great time. Time with patients in the exam rooms is precious, and the only reason I am still working. The patients are awesome!

Soon it was lunch time, and I'd seen all my morning patients. I went to the front desk and asked Jenna to take her lunch from 12 to 12:30, and then Agatha would go from 12:30 to 1 p.m.. That way, when patients arrived at 1 p.m., we'd have both ladies upfront greeting them. This met with Agatha's approval, which gave me another reason to go on living.

But at 12:30, Agatha was on the phone with Medicaid trying to get an ultrasound approval. The only reason Agatha was doing this was because she had cleared the ultrasound with the wrong provider, so she had to do it again.

I whispered, "Put the lady on hold." She ignored me.

Now getting more than a bit tense, I repeated, "Put the lady on hold."

Again, she ignored me. I had had enough.

I pushed the hold button myself.

Agatha gasped, shouting, "Doctor, why did you do that? I was talking to her!"

"Because I asked you to put her on hold three times and you didn't. Please take your lunch."

Agatha leapt to her feet and darted into the back room.

I got on the phone with the Medicaid rep and explained the situation, and she said that she understood. By then, Jenna was back and took over the phone call from me.

I headed back to my office, but on the way, as I passed my scheduler's office, I noticed Agatha in her office crying and complaining about me. During a previous dust-up Agatha created, I had her promise to come directly to me with any problems, rather than poison the well by griping to other employees.

I walked into my scheduler's office and asked, "What's going on?"

Agatha was on her feet. "I can't do this anymore! I'm drowning!"

Seriously, that's what she said. Drowning. Oh, the humanity. Agatha rushed to the front desk, grabbed her purse, and said she was clearing out right away.

Of course, that was when my first patient walked in for the afternoon; the woman quickly got a sense that Agatha was having a meltdown and was doing what she could to avoid my out-of-control front desk employee. I meekly told the patient that someone would be with her soon. Then I convinced Agatha to join me in my office. I didn't expect it to go well, but at least patients wouldn't enter my office to find an employee bawling her eyes out.

In my office, after we'd both taken a seat, I said, "What's going on? You were doing well yesterday. Today, you snapped at me and blew up because I was simply asking about everyday tasks. And you did it in front of patients, to boot. By the way, two of them mentioned it to me in the exam room. One of them asked how I could tolerate my staff speaking to me this way."

"I'm drowning!" she repeated. "I'm doing the work of three people!"

You would think she was working a pickax in a coal mine.

"We've always had one lady check people in, check them out, get charts ready, and during the 50 percent of the time we are not seeing patients, check faxes and referrals. I've taken 40 faxes, referrals, emails, and half of the charts away from you, and hired another full-time person to help you. I did that because you said you were doing the work of two people. So now you are doing the work of three people and am I supposed to hire another person? Next week, what happens if you decide that you're doing the work of four people? Or five?"

Agatha for once had nothing to say. At least I gave her credit for that, because any response would've been a complete BS and defensive gibberish.

I had to think of the practice and the other employees and the patients first. I pulled out every bit of managerial ingenuity I had ever read in a management book. So I spent 15 minutes telling Agatha how wonderful she was interacting with patients. I told her that her troubles often happened during down time, when patients weren't around. And then I praised her heartily for her ability to connect with the patients. There was truth to that part.

Then she reminded me that a bug had bitten her — I mean a literal bug, an insect – mosquito, sand fly, whatever, not a flu bug — and said it still hadn't gotten any better.

When she reached for the bite to scratch it, I told her that she would make it worse.

I dug a tube of Desitin out of my desk drawer and gave her some, telling her that this would "cure it."

As she applied the cream, I again reassured her that she was doing well at her job when it came to dealing with patients. I needed her to at least finish up the day until I could get a new lady up and running and hopefully deal with her drama and future on my time, not at my patients' expense.

"Can you finish the day now?" I asked her with as serious a face as I could muster.

She nodded.

The rest of the day went reasonably well, with Agatha coming up to me later and telling me, "Wow! My bug bite is almost gone!"

Her bug bite. Here she was in an office where clients often have cancer, and she thinks a bug bite is the end of the world.

Me? I just want to practice medicine. I don't want to be Dr. Phil, talking drama queens down from the ledge, or have to stroke egos just to keep people around for the rest of the day. But when you're running a medical practice, you have to play the role of coach, counselor, teacher, and boo-boo fixer because ultimately you have to get your staff to do their best for your patients as much as humanly possible.

I know that hiring issues are a challenge for a lot of professions. But doctors have to spend so much time cleaning up messes like this that they get distracted from the little quality time they have to take care of the patients.

It's essential for me to manage—and sometimes—bring to a finale—these employee and management challenges. Why? Because medicine is a people business and we care for others. Distracted and disenchanted employees hurt everything we do.

Productivity drops.

Complaining becomes contagious.

The other employees start to wonder whether I'm managing people under different sets of rules because I'm having to babysit one of them.

And the care of patients—and even the proper identification of patients—is put at risk.

I always want a strong, motivated and competent team around me—for my own sanity, yes, but especially for my patients!

Stories From The OR

When I'm performing surgery, I expect to control the process and quality of care that my patients receive. It's not about being a "control freak," but it is about doing everything I can to provide patients the best possible results, with the least likelihood of something going wrong.

Every surgeon has his or her own way of getting this done. And one day, I ran into a pair of issues that demonstrate how much I have to be on my toes, and how often I have to push back against those who might compromise a patient's care.

It was a Thursday afternoon, and after seeing patients in my private practice, I arrived at the hospital at lunchtime to do a double mastectomy with a sentinel lymph mode biopsy and bilateral reconstruction on a breast cancer patient. These surgeries are done jointly; as a breast cancer surgeon, I remove the breast and perform the lymph node biopsy, and then a plastic surgeon immediately follows with bilateral reconstruction.

As I came into the OR, I could see that the patient was already in the room and ready to be intubated. But I didn't recognize the young lady (okay, I'm not getting any younger, and more and more, new health care professionals looked to me like high school students) at the head of her bed but did know the CRNA next to her.

I said to the CRNA, "Is this the new young anesthesiologist?"

The CRNA whispered, "No, she is the anesthesia student."

"Wait a minute. Is she intubating my patient?"

CRNA nodded yes.

"No student should intubate my patients!" I said, stating a rule of mine that had been in place for several years at this hospital.

The CRNA said nothing.

"Where's the anaesthesiologist?" I asked.

I can't start the case until the patient is put to sleep, and the patient can't be put under until the anaesthesiologist comes into the room.

The CRNA shrugged.

So then it was up to me to hunt for the anaesthesiologist.

We were already delayed. So off I marched.

Eight years earlier, the anaesthesiology group, the only one allowed to work at this hospital, started training CRNA students for a fee. That meant that students, with no clearance or okay from the surgeons, would intubate the surgeon's patients. The intubation of my patients was tossed in like a free order of fries with their training—and the anaesthesiology group was benefitting for those fries.

We surgeons are the ones who make the decision to bring these patients to this hospital. The anesthesiologists have zero to do with that decision. And that patient cannot choose his or her anesthesiologist. In other words, anesthesiologists make a living when we surgeons decide to use this hospital for operations.

Part of my decision to use a community hospital is because I want my patients to have the confidence in knowing that residents or students will not be practicing or learning on them.

Keep in mind, anesthesiologists don't have to run an office, promote themselves, or get referrals, because they have an exclusive right to be the only anesthesiologist group that can work in the hospital. Also, the group in usually out of network, which means they get paid triple what the surgeon gets, many times at the expense of the patient's out of pocket amount due.

Yet they can increase their income by using our patients to have their students practice on them, and they get paid even more.

So when I noticed that my breast cancer patients were getting intubated by students, and after one student nearly ripped up my patient's vocal cords, I had enough. I went to the head of anesthesia.

"I'm not going to allow my patients to be intubated by a student again. I want it on my pre-op orders from now on."

"You can't do that. That's not your decision."

"Well, it is now. They're my patients. They don't know you and they come into surgery knowing that I brought them to a community hospital without students or residents."

We went back and forth for a while. I think he was surprised when I didn't back down. The wheels turned in his head, trying to decide whether this was a fight that was worth having. Ultimately, he agreed that the anesthesia department would not have students intubate my patients and got the OR committee to agree to the same.

Now, this wasn't good medicine or good management to give only me this out from student intubations. This was the department head's way to minimize how big a loss he was going to face. The safest policy would have been a hospital-wide rule that said students would not do intubations. Instead, he got the committee to approve a one-off policy created only for me. He wasn't going to allow other surgeons in the hospital to find out that was an option, because doing so might end his gravy train of being paid to teach students at a non-teaching hospital. Not only was this policy bad for everyone's patients except mine, but it was simply bad management.

You shouldn't lead a large health care company with so much money and so many lives at stake with different policies based on who the person is. In this case, I learned that when I spoke up, I got a policy changed. And I'm sure that other doctors who have complained about other things had policies created just for them. Having different rules for different people is a surefire way to create legal liability and angry employees.

Imagine what would happen if there was an intubation mistake made by a student that caused serious, even fatal, harm to a patient and a lawyer finds out that concerns about student intubations had been raised before, but not fully addressed.

Or for employees, how would you feel if your colleague gets preferential treatment, but you're stuck operating under the same old rules? That's a great way to turn a happy employee into a former employee.

After I spoke up, it was no surprise that the head of anesthesia made lots of complaints about me. I stepped on some toes that day and he couldn't resist retaliating against me.

But you know what? Tough! As the surgeon, it's my duty to make decisions that are in the best interest of my patients. Sure, I could take the easy way out, acquiesce, and agree to allow the anesthesiology group to use students or interns or some guy off the street to intubate. But I won't. And never will. If the anesthesiologists don't like me because of that, I can live with that.

It all comes down to this: When patients walk into the hospital, they're literally putting their lives in my hands. I don't take that lightly and, while training is acceptable and necessary, it's not appropriate for every situation.

But sometimes it's not about my ability to control the process during surgery. I have to rely on the staff. And most of the time, my confidence in the staff is rewarded. A current issue in this hyper-sensitive era where everyone is worried about microaggressions is that when a member of the surgical staff performs under par, any surgeon that brings the issue to the attention of administration could be subject to censure.

Think about that for a moment. Correcting someone whose actions could harm a patient may lead to a penalty for doing so.

Which brings me back to the double mastectomy.

The CRNA intubated the patient. So that was good for everyone—staff and patients.

Before we prep and drape patients, we typically inject 1 percent Lymphazurin blue dye into the patient's breast and massage it in for five minutes in order for the dye to travel to the hot sentinel lymph node, which is the one we are trying to remove and test. Basically, if it were a cancer cell, the dye would go to the lymph node first.

I asked the circulating nurse, "Do you have my syringe of Lymphazurin dye ready so I can inject into the patient?"

"Yes," she said.

She handed me a syringe full of blue dye. I injected it into the patient's breast and massaged.

The plastic surgeon came into the room and asked for his methylene blue dye, which he uses to outline the incisions and edges of the breasts.

The circulating nurse said, no kidding, "I just gave it to Dr. Nomine."

I was still massaging the dye into the patient's breasts. I said, "What?"

I looked over at her, whose eyes looked the size of silver dollars. She gulped audibly.

I said, "You just gave me methylene blue and not Lymphazurin?"

"Yes. Sorry, my mistake."

Yes, I thought, it certainly was your mistake.

My first reaction was to blow up. So many things can go wrong when somebody hands a surgeon the wrong syringe in the middle of surgery.

She asked me, "Do you want your Lymphazurin blue now to inject?"

"No!"

Despite the fact that we were already behind schedule due to having to hunt down the anesthesiologist earlier, I took a moment to think. Methylene blue takes a long time to get out of the skin and I was already worried about the mastectomy flap surviving with the methylene blue. I wasn't about to inject another blue dye. But I knew that some surgeons do use methylene blue to find the sentinel node, especially if the patient is allergic to Lymphazurin. So, the more I thought about it, the patient was going to be fine. Lucky. For all of us.

But I said, "You know that you need to double check what you're handing me. Did you know what was in the syringe you gave me?"

She said nothing. I would've preferred she acknowledged me and tell me this wouldn't happen again. Or something!

I'm happy to say that the surgery went well, despite the problems.

But the takeaway is this: I was waiting for the complaint that might come, stating that I had berated the OR staff or was rude or condescending toward the OR nurse. The frivolous complaints are taken as seriously as the legitimate ones and they can hurt you if you ignore them. And unfortunately, they also stop the ability to have important conversations. It's dangerous.

When we start to put feelings ahead of the patient's right to receive top quality health care with a minimum of mistakes, something has gone horribly wrong.

If behavior crosses into bullying and intimidation, that's one thing. But simply being direct when a life is at stake? Suck it up and have a grown-up conversation.

Hospital Protocol?

It was nine o'clock on a Friday morning when I discovered that some of my colleagues were full of crap.

I'm a surgeon, and I had performed a needle localization breast biopsy on a patient. That's one of those procedures that makes people cringe because it involves a long, thin wire plunged into breast tissue.

After I removed the specimen, there was a protocol to be followed. All hospitals have them, and ours was no exception. Accordingly, I sent the specimen to the radiology department for rapid x-raying while the patient remained, sedated, on the operating room table. This analysis takes about ten minutes, so the radiologist can confirm with the surgeon that the calcifications or mass detected on the mammogram has actually been removed.

I followed this protocol. Slavishly. Always did.

The radiologist didn't. His name was Dr. Hoffman, and the radiology department was only a few hallways down from the surgical suite. Arms crossed, I stood there, waiting in the operating room. And waiting.

Ten minutes. Twenty minutes.

I asked a nurse to locate Dr. Hoffman. She returned, wide-eyed, and reported Dr. Hoffman was nowhere to be found. I didn't want to risk anesthetizing the patient any longer than necessary.

The walls were closing in. I was Princess Leia stuck in the trash compactor.

I opted for the only logical course of action: wrap things up. I irrigated the wound, assured hemostasis and closed up, and they wheeled the patient out of the operating room into the recovery room. I busied myself with my other cases, while expecting to hear from Dr. Hoffman.

What the hell?

At noon, I called the radiology department and asked to speak with the elusive Dr. Hoffman.

"Oh, he already left for the day," the tech said. Really?

The radiologist tasked with calling me to provide the specimen's results … had skedaddled. I explained the protocol to the tech, though she certainly already knew, and requested that Dr. Hoffman call me immediately.

Six hours later, I had left the hospital and was in my car.

My cell phone rang.

"I hear you want to talk to me?" he asked, voice dripping with condescension.

"Dr. Hoffman, you never called me with the breast biopsy specimen radiograph result."

"Which one?" he said.

"Nine o'clock this morning."

I sensed him grappling for words. "I didn't know that I was supposed to call in the x-rays."

Dear God. That was a startling excuse, tantamount to his stating, "I'm incompetent."

"I have a hard time believing that," I remarked. "It's hospital protocol. Always has been."

"Well, you could've easily come down to Radiology to see the x-ray for yourself," he sputtered.

"Oh, please. I'm supposed to scrub out, walk down the hallway to look at an x-ray that you're supposed to read, then return and re-scrub to continue operating?"

Permit me to state the obvious. His prescribed plan of nonsense would have delayed the completion of the operation, which would have added to the patient's OR time, and their hospital bill, not to mention it would add more of a chance for infection. Plus, it's the job of the radiologist to read the specimen x-rays. He had been elaborately, extensively educated to do that and gets paid handsomely to do that. And not being a negligent chucklehead is part of the job description. And, worst of all, even if I read the x-ray, he would get paid as if he read it himself days after the fact.

There was something he wasn't telling me. I suspected he'd been snared by the temptations of male doctors everywhere: a girl or golf. But he wasn't saying.

We managed to end the call with a façade of cordiality.

But Dr. Hoffman hadn't apologized for anything.

Three days later, when I was in the office seeing patients, an x-ray report arrived via fax. It was the patient's specimen mammogram report from Dr. Hoffman. It revealed that the calcifications to be removed and tested were not in the specimen radiograph.

This case had ended around 9:15 am Friday. Dr. Hoffman submitted the specimen x-ray report on Monday morning, seventy-two hours later—and now it was too late to sample more breast tissue.

His report stated, "The specimen had no calcifications." In other words, he couldn't find the calcifications I was supposed to remove. I sighed and decided to wait for the pathology report. Said report presented the next day. The report stated the area was benign and there were microcalcifications in the pathology specimen. Thus, not only was the radiologist negligent in not reading the specimen's x-ray in a timely fashion, but he also read it incorrectly. He noted the calcifications were not in the specimen when they clearly were. That means Dr. Hoffman was wrong. Twice. However, the worst was yet to come.

Six weeks later, I received a letter from the hospital's quality assurance committee. This letter commented that I failed to reach the standard of care because I had not waited for the specimen's x-ray to be read. It also noted that I had not removed the calcifications because they had not been seen in the specimen x-ray.

In addition, the end of the letter noted I had been rude and spoken disrespectfully to Dr. Hoffman during the phone call in my vehicle.

That was, quite frankly, bull.

Immediately, I fired off a letter to the committee informing them that, when we removed the specimen, we sent it to the radiology department—per protocol—and waited for the radiologist to read it, per protocol, though he skipped out. More importantly, I laid out in clear, precise detail that not only was Dr. Hoffman stunningly late reading the x-ray on Monday morning, three days after the surgery, but further, he read it incorrectly.

Next afternoon, I went to speak to the head of the quality assurance committee. I stood in his office while he sat behind his desk and explained what happened.

"It's out of my hands," he said. "The matter was moved up to the MSQI committee."

I felt my breath catch in my throat. MSQI was the quality assurance committee for the entire hospital, not just the department of surgery. Worse, the head of the MSQI was Dr. Wells, a surgical ophthalmologist.

He was also my sworn enemy.

Years earlier, Dr. Wells attempted to prevent me from becoming chair of the surgical department by surreptitiously stacking the voting room with cronies who normally don't show up for surgical department meetings. This maneuver was designed to win more votes for himself. Nevertheless, I won and became chair of the department of surgery. He became vice chair, which pissed him off to no end. When my chairmanship ended, he succeeded me.

My concern was that he saw this event as some sort of Sicilian payback.

Dr. Wells also never missed an opportunity to thrust a non-compete agreement in someone's face for a signature. Later, he tried to enforce one against an ophthalmologist in his practice. I gave this particular poor soul the name of the attorney I'd hired to defend me against Dr. Wells' attempt to thrust a non-compete my way. They triumphed just as I did. I kept fighting because I didn't want this ridiculous situation to go on my record as faked evidence of my sinking standard of care.

Well, this fight went all the way to the MEC, the Medical Executive Committee, the pointy-headed, tippy-top of the medical pyramid.

Note that, usually, only severely negligent patient care goes all the way to the MEC. This committee is composed of the chairs of every department in the hospital—including the president of the medical staff, the chief medical officer, and the hospital's CEO.

It's like the Inquisition.

Worse, my name and reputation were endangered by merely appearing before the MEC.

I wore my crispest business outfit. In the meeting, I studied the array of individuals, many of whom were studiously avoiding eye contact with me.

I remember one of them asking if I had any questions.

That was the starting gun.

Bang, I was off.

"I have a question for the chair of the department of radiology," I said.

All eyes turned to me. The radiology chief shifted in his chair. "Go ahead," he said.

My voice came out sounding lower than a baritone sax. "I'd like to know," I said delicately, "why you haven't reprimanded Dr. Hoffman for not calling in that day."

He started to respond, but I interrupted. If I didn't say my peace now, I might be shut down. "And for not reading the specimen x-ray in a timely fashion? Dr. Hoffman didn't even look at it on the same day."

The chair opened his mouth to speak, but I still wasn't finished. "And why wasn't Dr. Hoffman reprimanded for reading the x-ray incorrectly?"

The radiology chair finally managed, "I have assessed the case, and I feel that Dr. Hoffman performed an adequate standard of care. He did nothing wrong."

And he said it with a straight face!

I sat there, wondering if he was waiting for Dr. Hoffman on the golf course that day. In fact, the entire department of radiology were business partners. Hence, it would be a conflict of interest for them to reprimand each other. They would all lose face and money if the hospital chose a different radiology group to have the exclusive rights to perform all radiology procedures in this hospital. The odds were stacked against me in a big way. But not in the department of surgery. We are all competitors. There's no incentive to support one's fellow surgeons.

If anything, there are incentives to reprimand each other.

I turned to the chair of the surgery department, Dr. Taylor. Earlier, he privately told me this was a witch hunt and I had done nothing wrong, so I knew he was on my side. Or so I thought.

"Dr. Taylor, what do you think about my decision to close up the patient instead of waiting until Monday for the report to come in?"

He cleared his throat, and his cheeks grew rosy. "You know, occasionally, I cover your calls when you're out of town."

"Yep," I said. "So?"

"So, that constitutes a conflict of interest."

"Meaning what?"

"Meaning, it's improper for me to give my opinion on whether you performed an adequate standard of care."

I was flabbergasted. This was a kangaroo court, and my one supposed ally had wimped out. If I had been an elderly woman, he was the good Samaritan who promised to help me cross the street, only to toss me under a passing Mack truck.

Maybe I shouldn't have been surprised. Remember, surgeons are competitors at this hospital, and Dr. Taylor was one of my main competitors. In fact, he and my husband often fought for the same operations. However, the radiology chair was a direct business partner of Dr. Hoffman, and he'd felt zero conflict of interest in absolving the radiologist of wrongdoing. He also was the instigator of the complaint against me for being "rude" to the radiologist.

I don't like to play the woman card, but I wonder if I would've received the same complaint if I were a man. I bet by raising my voice I would've been deemed passionate instead of rude.

I wasn't the only person weirded out by this farce. The other internal medicine doctors—the non-surgeons—in the room appeared quite uncomfortable. They could see something didn't look right. But none would speak up on my behalf. I turned back to Dr. Taylor. "So, I should've waited in the operating room the entire weekend? I should've not closed up the patient for seventy-two hours?"

Dr. Wells chimed in. "Enough with the hyperbole."

I'll halt the hyperbole when Dr. Hoffman stops playing hooky with his little side piece! I wanted to say, before restraining myself.

The meeting ended with my restating my overall professionalism. I noted that my patient had experienced an excellent outcome, despite Dr. Hoffman's inadvertent efforts to sabotage the operation.

Patient health is always the main objective. I achieved it. Do no harm.

I left the room and stomped back to my office. I didn't care if Dr. Hoffman was reprimanded. All I wanted was a just conclusion—that I did nothing wrong and that I didn't perform below the standard of care.

The MEC's letter arrived on the morning of the third day.

I opened it with shaking hands.

My eyes widened as I drank in the dry, bureaucratic prose. The medical executive committee had deemed me to have not performed up to the standard of care. I felt the built-up pressure rising within me.

Two hours later, another letter arrived. It, too, was from the MEC. I ripped this one open. The second letter stated that the decision was made to deem this case "no-fault."

Which meant I wasn't innocent but wasn't guilty. To this day, I don't know who made the decision. There's a special place in heaven waiting for the anonymous and decent individual who intervened to make that happen.

But I have my own theory about what happened.

Dr. Hoffman knew I would most likely complain about his unprofessionalism. Consequently, he proceeded to complain about me to the chair of the radiology department (a.k.a. his business partner) before I could lodge my own complaint, which of course I never had any intention of doing. Frankly, I'm too busy.

My main point is I'm a female private practice surgeon going up against the Boys Club with a complicated web of conflicts of interest. Yet they got to use the term *in the best interest of the patient* as an excuse to make my life miserable. They steamrolled and smeared me, hoping I would either quit or that referral doctors would no longer send patients to me, thereby running me out of business.

What they didn't realize is they picked the wrong girl to fight with. When I'm right, I don't back down. Or give up and run away like a scolded child. They targeted a surgeon who believes in herself and what's best for her patients and knows it's a waste of time to get involved with the political hospital drama.

After all, the shady parts of modern medicine divert me from my only goal: to take care of my patients to the very best of my abilities.

Some health care professionals forget that. Not me.

I don't care about breaking some eggs if it means I provide the best possible patient care. And they thank me for this.

Nothing else matters.

Wrong Number

I was doing a Needle localization/lumpectomy with Sentinel Lymph Node Biopsy.

I said to the circulating nurse (that's a nurse who is in charge of preparations for an operation), "Have a pathologist look at the sentinel lymph node to see if it cancerous."

She called pathology. But fifteen minutes later, no pathologist had arrived.

I said to the circulating nurse, "Can you call again?" She nodded, walked off and called again.

When she returned, she said, "They're on their way."

But we waited and no pathologist. "Did you call another hospital mistakenly?"

"Nope," she said.

"Okay. We have to do something. Will you call the front desk and have them call pathology?"

Turns out, that my circulating nurse had been calling another hospital's pathologist, who was not the pathologist on this case. So of course the pathologist thirty minutes away went to the OR in his hospital looking for a specimen that was not there. Because it was in a completely different hospital!

When the correct pathologist finally did arrive, he said, "Odd that she didn't know how to make the call correctly."

"True," I said. "But it isn't my job to train staff on how to call the hospital where we are actually located and not the hospital thirty minutes away. I'll leave that to the OR administration or they will say something about me overstepping my bounds or making trouble or being rude to somebody or other."

The pathologist nodded. "True. Sad, but true."

Friday Morning Bouts: Radiologist Smack Down

Friday, my busiest operating day.

I had four operations. One of them was a needle localization lumpectomy, which involved removing suspicious clusters of calcifications from my patient's breast.

But before I could do anything, the patient needed to go into radiology, in order to get a needle/wire placed into the area of the breast containing the calcifications that I would later remove and test for cancer.

But I got a surprise. I was told there were no needle localizations being done on Fridays anymore.

To which I responded, "What?"

I was told that the radiology group has decided they will no longer do needle localizations on Friday. And further told me that an email weeks or months before from the head of radiology let me know about the new policy.

Time for a little back story.

When I earlier mentioned, "the" radiology group working, I meant just that. One radiology group. So we can't just call in another radiologist because this radiology group has what's called an exclusivity agreement with the hospital. Your standard monopoly. Why is this so? I don't understand it. Competition is good.

This hospital is a full-service hospital: a trauma center, a cancer center, but for some reason it was decided that we would have zero radiology coverage to perform a very common surgical procedure on Fridays.

By comparison, if surgeons refused to perform a consultation or operation or were somehow unavailable for whatever reason, the referring doctor or patient could request another surgeon. But we surgeons and doctors, who I would like to think are kind of important when it comes to surgical procedures, don't have the same right when it comes to radiologists refusing to perform a service for us.

I went to the OR managing nurse and asked her why this policy was agreed to. She didn't know.

So I called the head of the OR committee. She looked into it and informed me that the COO of the hospital okayed the radiologists' wishes to not do needle localizations on Fridays. Since Friday is my main operating day, this was infuriating and harmful to my patients.

She contacted the radiology group, who asked why I could not just perform needle localizations on Monday through Thursday?

I responded that my patients often request their operations on Fridays, because that way they can only take one day off from work and then recover over the weekend. Changing my OR to accommodate radiologists significantly inconvenienced my patients.

Getting back to the heart of the matter, you may well ask why can't any radiologist, like any surgeon, cardiologist, etc., get privileges to practice at the hospital?

If you get an answer on that, make sure I'm the first to know!

One Scrub Short

My husband was about to perform a bowel resection. He had requested a second scrub. This is standard operations for a resection, and any operation. But just as he got started, he was told the hospital did not have enough staff to help with the operation.

Not surprisingly, he was struggling, and had his staff call me to come and help. I rushed over.

Once there, I realized they still had no staff available to provide a second scrub. A scrub tech came in, but only to ask the scrub tech on duty if she needed a break. Which meant the hospital did not have the staff to help the surgeon during a major operation, but apparently did have staff enough to ensure that everyone got breaks. Also, several staff members who could've helped in the OR were just standing around in front of the OR scheduling board. Some explained that they had meetings to go to, whatever that means.

This is where culture matters. In some hospitals, employees would have looked at the problem and pitched in to fill the void. Here, they tried to blend into the wall to avoid doing work.

So I ask you: did patient care come first? I certainly don't think so.

I believe that any patient having a colon resection would consider this a serious operation, want the best of care, and want a full staff.

But for those who forget what made them want to become a doctor in the first place, decisions to operate (literally) at less than the best of levels occurs far too often.

I must mention that there are a few staff members who actually do come in on their days off to help surgeons, including me, by serving as a second scrub when they know the hospital won't assign a second. A sincere thanks to those people – you know who you are!

Pregnant Pause

I waited for my first patient of the day at 8:00 a.m. The surgery was slated for 8:30 a.m. Mind you, the patient arrived at the hospital 5:30 a.m. The patient was "blue hat" ready at 8:15 a.m. But I learned that the pregnancy test that the preop nurse had sent at 5:30 a.m. not only had not been reviewed until 8:20 a.m., but the test needed to be repeated.

Of course, this caused a delay. And the pregnancy test requires urine, which the patient was unable to produce at that point. Had the test been checked any time before 8:20 a.m., it could have been repeated, but because it wasn't, the surgeon, the patient, the OR staff, and the anesthesiologist (whose license would've been at stake without a pregnancy test) were all stuck waiting.

I asked the pre-op nurse why the test wasn't checked long before that point.

I was told, "I don't know." Sigh.

I didn't bother complaining to the preop nurse, and instead kicked it upstairs to an administrator, who at least said, "Thanks. This should not have happened and we're looking into it."

Better than nothing, I guess.

This is all a great example of how too much in health care gets caught up in 'this is how we've always done it' type of thinking. Instead of solving problems that effect everyone, we all protect our little piece of territory. This inhibits success.

Too much of health care prides itself as being better and different than the business world, but we can learn things from streamlined, cohesive operations that search for processes that ensure consistently positive outcomes and efficiency.

In this example, why couldn't safety have occurred at 5:30, 6:30 or even 7:30? One department's selfishness and singular focus delayed us all. Why must we be "safe" after the OR case is supposed to start? In other words, why is ineptitude disguised as patient safety?

And why are huge patient delays caused by professional ineptness and rudeness treated as an acceptable casualty in the treatment process?

We have software that addresses every possible staff and productivity issue except the one that might make the experience better for our patients.

Imagine the improvement that could come with an approach that began with wanting to address a patient's needs in a way that looks at the whole customer experience from beginning to end—and decide the goal is to make them well, but also make them as satisfied as possible.

People understand delays, but the feeling among our health care professionals that our time matters more than that of our patients is a glaring weakness in the system. Change that and you improve conditions overnight! Why? Because we're creatures of habit and we get comfortable in our habits. When we get too comfortable, we get lazy and careless. Occasional bad actions become habits. When it comes to the respect of other people's time, it's been forgotten. And for those making investments in health care, there is a huge opportunity ahead for medical professionals who treat people with care—and respect for their schedules and treating them like a valued customer.

Healing Doctors

You've heard the saying *Play the hand you're dealt.*

It means you take on the challenge that's sitting right in front of you because you really don't have a choice.

When it comes to healing the doctors within our system, it means doctors owning the mistakes they make, but also means dealing with a system that often puts paperwork before patients and drives doctors out of the profession.

It also involves doctors trying to succeed in a system that squeezes their ability to make the salary required to pay off the average $195,000 in student loan debt that doctors carry into their first job.

And it means many doctors have to fight through their lack of strong communication skills to provide outstanding customer care.

Finally, in other cases, we see burnout among doctors skyrocketing and it's created a climate where doctors decide between continuing in a system they can't stand any longer or changing careers. I've felt it! The paperwork and having to answer to my boss who does not pay me one dime in salary (the insurance company pays me) is what causes the burnout that I occasionally feel. There are, however, ways to connect doctors back to what brought them into medicine in the first place—helping patients.

Putting Patients Over Paperwork Again

Our health care system prioritizes paperwork over people. It's that simple.

I'm going to show you exactly how much the system incentivizes that backwards thinking, show you the problem, and then encourage amazing doctors to find a way to fight through the busywork trap that is creating a barrier between them and patients.

A study by Christine Sinsky, MD, of the American Medical Association followed and requested feedback from 57 doctors across the spectrum from family medicine to specialists. What Sinsky found was predictable but alarming: that is, doctors spend most of their time doing paperwork.

Sinsky's study showed doctors spend:

+ 27% of their time seeing patients
+ 49.2% of their time doing paperwork

I think doctors may be embarrassed to talk about how much paperwork they actually do, as I find that I see patients 10 percent of the time with the other 90 percent spent doing paperwork, administrative duties and fighting over billing issues with insurance companies.

But regardless of the exact number for each doctor, Sinsky's numbers demonstrate further than even when the doctors are in the exam rooms with patients, it didn't mean doctors and patients are communicating. In fact, Sinsky's research shows that even when doctors are in the room with their patients, they spend 37.9 percent of their time doing paperwork and just over half the time talking to or examining patients. This is why I refuse to bring my computer into the exam room.

If you're wondering whether this is just a rant about a dislike of paperwork, know the following: Doctors are mandated by law to do it.

Electronic Medical Records (EMR) requires the following to be filled out for each patient:

- administrative and billing data
- patient demographics
- progress notes
- vital signs
- medical history
- diagnoses

- medications
- immunizations
- allergies
- radiology images
- lab and test results

Regulations require a doctor to personally enter much of this information for accuracy reasons, which can cut down on prescription errors. But imagine the time a doctor is spending on the keyboard in front of elderly patients who likely are suffering from 2 or 3 chronic illnesses simultaneously! So when your doctor is spending time doing data entry instead of checking your pulse, there's a bureaucrat, insurance company or politician somewhere who is demanding it!

And it's not because they care about the patient. It's about billing and making sure that as little money as possible flows to doctors. The insurance companies aren't in the business of regulating proper levels of care because that's not their business.

And the worst part is that EMR requirements are getting worse every day, as state regulations, insurance requirements, and other informational mandates pile up.

EMR requirements also provide false assurances of accuracy and complete information. Doctors inserting ten pages of information about a patient's diagnosis may be useful information—or it may be incoherent rambling.

The requirement for electronic medical records was sold to the American public and elected officials as easy access to information, quick transfer from one doctor to another, an informational bonanza for use in emergency situations, and a simplification of a complicated web of old, dusty file cabinets of information from throughout the medical system.

What we got instead is a time-sucking productivity drag on doctors that doesn't do nearly enough for patients in return. Insurance companies and EMR companies worked together to dupe our elected officials.

What's the solution? It won't be easy, but doctors need to turn away from their computer screens and spend an extra moment or two to connect with patients and let them know that they are the top priority. Maybe we can start to each take a note or two about what's happening in the patient's life, put it into our personal notes, and ask about it at the next appointment. That type of attention may make all the difference in the quality of life for our patients on their future medical visits—and for doctors!

The biggest irony of EMRs is that they don't provide better patient care. It's worse because doctors don't have as much time to spend with their patients due to all the time they're entering data into the computer. Data inputting can and does have as many errors as the paper forms.

The second myth about electronic medical records is that they're more private. You know, HIPAA? Well, that's false too. It's much easier for someone to hack into a computer file than go into my office and find a chart that is organized by numbers and not names. So there are two bogus claims by our government and special interest groups who lobby for these laws (so that they can make money off of doctors and patients). I tell my patients that however long you see me in this room with you, multiply that amount of time by ten and that is the amount of time I actually spend on you. So, five minutes in the room with you means I've spent 50 minutes entering information editing your notes, sending your bill with the proper mandated insurance codes, fixing any errors that the insurance company always finds even when there aren't any, sending additional records requested by the insurance company before they will pay the claim(knowing that 50 percent of doctor's offices will not send the records and therefore absolving the insurance company from paying a dime) and time discussing your case with your referring doctor and/or faxing the note to the referring doctor. Whew! I work from 5pm to 12am every weeknight typing up my notes in my EMR getting charts ready for the next day so I can see my patients in a timely manner. After I've seen my patients, I then spend three more hours a day in my office finishing the notes I started the night before. Then on the weekends I spend four hours Saturday and four hours Sunday getting my charts ready for Monday, reviewing the charges from the previous week and reconciling the deposits from the 5 previous days. So if medicine was just actually taking care of patients, I would love it and would want to do it forever, but it is basically a secretary job with a MD title requiring 14 years (in my case) extra training after high school.

What's lost in that time of paper pushing? Important time with our patients, a resting of our minds and energies on the occasional free weekend, professional development, and the extra time to build stronger teams within our staffs. Patients will benefit if balance is found allowing doctors back into their role as provider of care, not full-time data entry clerk.

If balance is created, patients will be the big winners. They'll receive more personalized care and focused doctors who are currently left wondering how they became data entry clerks.

The REAL Practice of Medicine:

Here's how it works in the American medical system today for new doctors:

1. A baby-faced, idealistic medical student studies non-stop, has no social life outside of their classes, excels on their tests, and after years of no sleep and long residencies, graduates with a world of excitement, success, and an average of nearly $200,000 in student loan debts in hand.

2. They then have to go through three to seven years of residency depending on their specialty at barely minimum wage. So that's even more years stuck in a building while others are living their lives, starting families etc.

3. They move into a relatively high-paying job upon residency graduation, but the job turns their lives into an endless series of mini-appointments driven by spectacularly limited reimbursement rates set by the federal government and insurance companies, not lifechanging moments they dreamed of when they decided they wanted to become a doctor.

The average doctor sees 20 patients per day and works 51 hours per week in the office—not including whatever they bring home with them. Most doctors work far more than this, as our instinct to be a dedicated care provider pushes most of us way past those averages. That works out to two patients per hour for 10 hours per day, with much of that time jammed with paperwork, answering questions and requests from staff, an understandable need for a minute or two to decompress from the previous appointment and any briefings before the new appointment.

How does a patient-focused doctor emerge from that rat race? How do positive patient outcomes consistently come from that much commotion and so little patient contact and true interaction? It's a credit to the amazing doctors who dedicate their lives to serving others and the amazing staffs around them who provide great service to their patients, but I am a firm believer that our health care system must demand better for everyone who enters a doctor's office.

Why? Patients still respect the profession of medicine in study after study, but patients are also taking note of how many doctors are chained to their computer like a bunch of gamers, and they aren't happy about it.

Again, I do not bring computers into the room with a patient. I take notes and then enter data later. Eye contact and one on one experience with people at difficult times in their lives matters—and it builds trust. Does it mean I spend more time entering information later in the day? Oh yes. But it's worth it.

But not every doctor will sacrifice that extra time later in the day. For those that won't, there are some ways to humanize the process more.

In a 2011-2013 study, researchers from the University of California, San Francisco, studied interaction between 47 patients and 39 doctors at a public hospital. Researchers determined how much doctor's computer use occurred in each appointment. The appointments with high computer usage were rated as excellent approximately half the time. Nearly 80 percent of the low computer use appointments were rated "excellent."

So, if patients hate the computer usage and the doctors don't like it either but are required to be chained to it by law, what's the solution?

And, with government calling the shots on patient interaction, can solutions even be implemented?

Indiana University School of Medicine professor Richard Frankel, PhD, is a medical sociologist who studied exam room computer use and then interviewed patients after the fact.

He states that computers have been a part of doctor's offices for 25-30 years, but now likens them to almost a third person in the room because of their significant role in every visit.

Via a federal grant, Frankel developed a way to help diminish patient frustration with technology overload. It's called POISED, a series of best practices that gets patients and doctors talking and best of all explains why doctors seem to be putting keyboards over conversations.

- Prepare—Doctors should review patient records before seeing a patient whenever possible. I do this in the evenings prior to the patient's appointment.

- Orient—Explain to patients during an exam how the computer use plays a role in health care and how some of it benefits them. Doctors can also use that time to get valuable feedback from patients

- Information—enter information from patients in realtime, as once you have instructed patients about the importance of data, you do not want to diminish it by your actions.

- Share—turn the computer screen, so the patient can see what has been typed.

- Educate—use the computer as a teaching tool with patients where possible and use it as the basis for conversation that helps the patient understand their health better and any instructions they may need to hear.

- Debrief—use the discussions and the computer information to reinforce any direction they need. Many times after I visit with my patient in the exam room.

I will bring them into my office and go over their information, pathology etc. while we both look at their chart in my computer. This is my way of making sure I don't miss anything and the patient is fully informed of their health and care.

I have so far refused to take my computer into my patient's room. I instead write what I typed into the computer and bring it in to the room. This, of course, triples my work. Type it, write it, update the writing, update the typing. To me, the extra work is worth giving my patients' eye contact and conversation.

Even so, computers aren't going to leave exam rooms anytime soon, but the more doctors who can turn them into a positive or at least explain the use of them away, the better! And, at the very least, it makes people understand that their doctor isn't disinterested in them or obsessed with screentime—it's that they're mandated by law to enter this information. The sooner more patients—especially those who know their elected officials—understand that, the better!

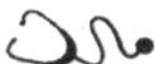

What else can doctors do to promote a process that helps patients, but also makes them feel more connected? Be a good listener, don't judge when asking questions, and ask open-ended questions that can prompt better discussion and more helpful information.

In her book, *What Patients Say, What Doctors Hear*, Dr. Danielle Ofri says doctors need to communicate better and drive out opinions and bias from their questions. Citing research showing bias against patients with obesity as an example, Ofri suggests that doctors think about whether their questions are really questions—or more like editorials. Also, Ofri urges doctors to avoid interruptions that can shut down good doctor-patient discussion, noting a University of South Carolina study showing that patients are often interrupted within 12 seconds of beginning their comments to a doctor. Listen for content and understanding, not to just lead into the next question. Ofri also suggests that doctors ask patients, "Is there anything else?" before ending the appointment. That may open up a long line of discussion with a few patients, but it may also detect something important that a patient had previously never revealed.

Burnout Battles

Doctor burnout is real.

You've just read all about the daily hamster wheel-like existence of doctors, but you've also learned some ways doctors can turn frustrating constraints into rewarding experiences.

But burnout, which can come from the day-to-day frenetic pace, can hurt everyone. The signs are obvious, and much the same for burnout in any profession:

- Emotional exhaustion that simply going home and resting doesn't solve.
- Disconnection from others that manifests itself in lack of ability to communicate effectively with patients and criticism of others.
- Lack of confidence that leads to feeling that a doctor is not accomplishing anything important.

There are many ways to deal with burnout, ranging from talking to other doctors who have been there to finding ways outside of work that allow them to decompress from their stressful daily lives.

Burnout detection should also come from fellow doctors. When we see it, we need to encourage doctors to get rest and get an attitude adjustment before it seriously affects patients. Carelessness, even the accidental type, kills.

And when doctors see other doctors who are becoming reckless, abusive and doing harm to their people and patients, we need to step up and respond too.

Addressing the challenges we have discussed is only one part of the equation. Hospital and health systems need to be cured of their problems also.

Healing Hospitals and Health Care Systems

Hospitals and the systems that manage them are among the most vital and fast-changing components of the health care sector, but also the most challenging to fix. The challenges are complex, expensive, and often controversial.

And it's for all of those reasons that they must be cured of what ails them.

The organizational culture of hospitals is one of the biggest challenges and opportunities facing health care. Culture can be a magnet to attract the best of the best, but also repel people out of individual hospitals and even the medical profession.

A December 2019 article in the *Journal of American Physicians and Surgeons* blames a wide range of symptoms that lead to burnout, all pointing to cultural problems that become operational policy—whether people acknowledge it or not.

They include the following:

- Administrative punishment for noncompliance with select organizational policies and objectives
- Informal punishment (through whisper campaigns and lack of promotions)
- Scapegoating of certain employees when things go wrong
- The substitution of legal and administrative standards for professional standards
- Risk management geared towards institutional interests over those of patients and doctors
- Peer reviews that appear geared toward pre-judged outcomes

Every one of those actions makes the health care system weaker, because when trust breaks down, the system breaks down.

Battling the Bullies in Health Care

A 2016 Occupational Safety and Health Administration (OSHA) report put a spotlight on exactly how prevalent bullying is in health care and how damaging it is to health care outcomes. Focusing on nursing, it said 21 percent of nurses and nursing students reported being physically assaulted and over half were verbally abused in the last year. For emergency nurses alone, 12 percent said they experienced physical violence and 59 percent faced verbal abuse in the last seven days!

Bullying comes from all directions and is defined as repeated, health-harming mistreatment by one or more perpetrators.

Bullying manifests itself through isolation, sabotage, threats to professional status, insults and name calling, and overwork.

In a health care setting, 44 percent of nurses say they've been bullied and much of it, as the OSHA study showed, comes from nurse-on-nurse bullying. It's the reason there's a saying "nurses eat their own!" As you're reading these things, I'm sure you feel compassion for the nurse, doctor or anyone else that is bullied. None of us want to go through that, but there's another victim to bullying when it happens in health care—the patient.

When you look at the tactics used by bullies, the most dangerous ones for patients are isolation, sabotage and overwork. Isolation usually takes the form of cutting someone off from information flows. In other words, withholding valuable information. In health care, that type of secrecy can be fatal if someone does not have the right information when they need it. Sabotage can occur in many different ways, but it can easily affect a patient's outcomes through a professional being distracted or mistrusting of the information they've been given. Finally, overwork is common in health care, as I can readily attest to, but purposeful overwork by an abusive boss can reach a level where the employee hits a breaking point—which is the intended goal of a bully. This is where life and death mistakes can happen—that is, when people are exhausted or become rattled to the point of not being at a safe level of competency.

The effects on the individual are clear, but it affects patients too. According to the Joint Commission, "Workplace bulling leads to lawsuits, compensation for disability, loss of profits, negative impact on organizational reputation and a corrosion of the patient to health care worker relationship."

Also, it's no shock that safety and quality concerns mount. Why? A bullied employee becomes much less likely to want to speak up for any reason for fear of continued targeting.

Common decency and respect aren't a lot to ask from medical professionals, but unfortunately too many people at all levels of medicine are falling short. We can do better!

When hospital cultures go bad, especially in high pressure areas like emergency rooms, they're tough to fix and the risks are high.

Why? If there's a toxic culture within a group, it is usually imposed by or ignored by the top of the organization.

When you consider that toxic behaviors often include the inability to discuss tough problems, low employee feedback, and retaliation, you have a recipe for disaster for patients in times of crisis or when mistakes are made. Why? People are afraid to speak up if mistakes are made by people—whether by those in power or at lower levels who are in fear of losing their jobs. This type of atmosphere can literally cost lives.

It causes too many medical professionals to mind their own business and avoid looking out for problems they see around them.

The shocking and infamous case of Dr. Death, the former neurosurgeon Christopher Duntsch, shows why doctors must always protect patients and the profession over any individual doctor.

But it also speaks to the weaknesses that exist in a health care system that seems to lack either the infrastructure, the processes or the will to screen out its bad actors.

Duntsch became a surgeon in Texas in 2010 and almost immediately began to maim patients in 33 surgeries across multiple hospitals, including:

- severed an artery in a patient's spine, causing them to bleed to death
- cut another patient's vertebral artery causing a massive, fatal stroke

- damaged nerve roots during a spinal fusion surgery, and left surgical tools inside the patient
- mistook a neck muscle for a tumor, severed a vocal cord, cut a hole in the esophagus, and left a surgical sponge in a throat—all in one surgery!

While Duntsch was fired by a series of hospitals, he continued to move from hospital to hospital in Texas until two concerned doctors, Randall Kirby and Robert Henderson, spoke out and called for Duntsch's medical license be revoked. While eventually successful in getting his license revoked, Kirby and Henderson feared Duntsch moving on to cause destruction in another state. They urged the Dallas County District Attorney's Office to charge Duntsch criminally, saying they could produce evidence that Duntsch planned to intentionally hurt his patients. Their efforts were successful, and in 2015, Duntsch was charged with 11 counts of assault with a deadly weapon and one count of injury to a child, elderly or disabled person.

In 2017, Duntsch was convicted and sentenced to life in prison.

But it only got fixed because two doctors were willing to speak up and call attention to a colleague who was harming their patients. In an industry often reluctant to address its issues, Drs. Kirby and Henderson are heroes.

But a weakness of the system emerged in the Duntsch case from the fact that Duntsch was able to find job after job as a surgeon in his area despite having begun his reign of terror. Was anyone within these health care systems checking references or were they simply relying on his status as a doctor for all the credentials that they needed?

Beyond the cultural problems described here, our hospitals and health care systems are daily repeating common mistakes that cause unnecessary money to be spent and time that is wasted on procedures that benefit no one except medical professionals, the systems and occasionally the convenience of patients.

A 2012 study published in the *Journal of the American Medical Association* (JAMA) found that between one-third and one-half of all medical costs are due to overuse of diagnostic tests, therapeutic procedures, and medications.

Additionally, out of concern about the aggressive litigation environment in which we live, defensive medicine is alive and well. Defensive medicine is health care practiced in ways that reduce litigation risk, usually done through the use of excessive diagnostic testing.

The estimates of the cost of defensive medicine vary from $45 billion up to $200 billion annually—all for the purpose of avoiding a lawsuit.

Some of the concerns about litigation manifest themselves in health care system procedures, as doctors are encouraged to provide testing that reduces legal risk.

An August 2019 *Journal of the American Medical Association* (JAMA) report showed that the rate of certain diagnostic tests being run by peers of a doctor reported for malpractice jumped by nearly 50 percent for a short period of time after the filing.

The ripple effect on a peer-to-peer basis is understandable.

As all politics is local, so is everything else.

There are other major concerns that hospitals and systems must face, as the health care consumer is demanding it. They include:

+ Find ways to make the patient feel like they're receiving individualized care specifically for them.

+ Figure out ways to bring doctors closer to the patient experience, not push us further away. With the paperwork burdens I've discussed with EMRs, can technology take away some of the time paperwork fills up?

Defensive Medicine is Offensive

Defensive medicine is both completely understandable and completely unacceptable. For very different reasons.

Defensive medicine at the most basic level is usually defined as medicine that's practiced to avoid malpractice litigation, but it's just as often used to fight against the concern that we could be wrong—or do not want to disappoint the family of the patient sitting in front of us.

According to a 2013 study by Jackson Health care, one of the largest health care staffing agencies in the U.S., 75 percent of doctors say they order more procedures, tests, and medicine than might be necessary—all to avoid lawsuits. In other words, it's a cover your bases strategy that likely reduces risk but explodes costs.

Gallup has reported that one in four dollars spent—or nearly $700 billion!—can be attributed to defensive medicine. Defensivemedicine.org puts that number at $850 billion, while some sources attribute defensive medicine as a negligible cost. Why? Because in theory, any test that a doctor orders can be justified by someone. However, ask the same doctor about their colleague's over-testing and you'll get lots of hot opinions about how necessary some of those tests are. In other words, the standards are there for thee, not for me! You'll never hear anyone admit they're doing it. But because of the risk of not doing it, they're doing it.

Every doctor has met the patients who use WebMD and other medical websites like it's a medical diagnosis.

They type symptoms like headaches and sore throats and get back answers that tell them they may have anything from allergies to brain tumor to Covid-19. When patients become unglued with the possibility of that range of maladies, some doctors give in to their fears instead of seriously applying medicine. We let them have what they want instead of what they need.

It's maddening and, in our efforts to rule out problems, many doctors take the easy way out and over-prescribe, over-test, and generally overdo it. We cater to the concerned family members who want "whatever it takes" to be used to combat what may or may not be a serious issue, may have a very simple, identifiable solution, or sadly may be too late. Also, lots of doctors are nervous about bad online ratings, so they'll gladly order additional, unnecessary tests that they may not think are necessary, if it means they avoid a bad review.

Additionally, there are financial incentives when conducting additional tests, which further clouds the thinking.

What's fascinating in so many of the findings about defensive medicine is that some doctors—for both reasonable as well as silly reasons—have lost confidence in their ability to manage their patients well. In 2005, a study by Studdert and published in the *Journal of the American Medical Association*, found that 92 percent of doctors admit to ordering imaging tests and diagnostic measures for assurance and 42 percent were eliminating high risk procedures and avoiding patients with significant complications. That's a lot of doctors who appear to not be able to either make a strong decision or fear doing so.

In addition to the financial damage to the system, beyond the costs that everyone pays for through increased premiums to help pay for the wasteful procedures, there are patient specific risks, including:

+ radiation exposure
+ bleeding and infection from biopsies
+ through overuse of some antibiotics, patients can lose their ability to fight off some viruses.

Trial attorneys are another sector that create generational wealth on the backs of doctors and patients. Why should a patient who had died or had a complication of treatment (even if the fault of the doctor) provide millions of dollars of income to an attorney? That money should go to the family or patients only. And if an appendix removal is worth $500 if done correctly, why is it worth three million dollars if something goes wrong? Why out of that three million dollars does the attorney get over a million?

The Cost of Insane Pricing

Can anyone in health care explain to a reasonably smart person health care pricing, such as:

- Why IV bags costs approximately $1, but are billed by some hospitals as high as $546?
- Or why a Band-Aid, and its accompanying service fee, totals $629?
- Or why an aspirin costs an ER patient $30?
- Or why treating a sprained ankle can cost anywhere from $4 to $24,000?
- Or why you can be charged $200 per minute for time in the emergency room?

Of course none of this makes sense, but there are literally thousands of similar pricing anomalies that exist through-out the health care system. Why? Because if we knew the actual cost of procedures in the health care marketplace, we would immediately see more price competition.

There are efforts to create competition in health care that are getting people's attention and their health care business.

One of those is the Surgery Center of Oklahoma, a multi-specialty state-of-the-art facility in Oklahoma City. Owned by 40 surgeons around the Sooner State, the SCO is ideal for health care customers with the increasingly frequent high-deductible insurance plans, but also employees who work for self-insured companies.

A quick glance on their site shows that an Achilles tendon repair costs $5,730, which is all-inclusive. Arthroscopic knee surgery costs $3,740 all-in.

But just try asking a surgeon at any other hospital in the country that question. You would be checked for a concussion for even asking!

To be fair, there are many factors that go into the price of a procedure. The diagnostic tools (and the cost for the use of them), the medications, the use of the OR, the cost for each of the specialists involved in a surgery will vary greatly, as can the post-op care, recovery room cost and any potential overnight stays in a room. And even with all of these variables, so many other costs are loaded into other parts of the bill, most medical professionals have no idea of the full cost of anything other than their particular role. I don't know that it was purposefully designed to confuse, but the result has become mass pricing confusion.

With all of this apples-to-oranges pricing in health care, it's confusing, but most people won't ask questions about price for another reason: insurance.

Insurance ensures that we no longer worry about the price. People care up to the point they hit their deductible and then the concern often ends. But insurances deductibles will just continue to rise. Remember, insurance companies always win.

Here's a novel idea: how about I ask my patient to get authorizations directly from her insurance company when they are acting up about covering her operation?

I had a patient with newly diagnosed breast cancer. We scheduled her for L breast needle localization lumpectomy with L sentinel lymph node biopsy. Her insurance was Humana.

Following the usual procedure, my staff called Humana to get the authorization codes for the outpatient surgery (my patient would go home the same day). Typically, the lymph node biopsy codes did not require prior authorization. But in this case, the insurance rep told my staff that we did require prior authorization, and that we would need to get that code that by calling a different phone number. Okay, a time suck, as my staff had already spent an hour on the phone about this, but no worries.

We did as we were told and were instructed that it would take six days to get this authorized. My patient's surgery was scheduled in 10 days, so, so far so good. Or you might think. With my patient's surgery scheduled on a Thursday, my staff called the Friday before, only to learn that there was a denial on the lumpectomy code, instructing us that we needed to do a peer-to-peer consult with the insurance company's medical director, who would need to approve it. This was a first.

My scheduler set up the appointment and gave me the insurance doctor's phone number. I called him at the anointed time. No answer. I left a voicemail asking for a call back and told him why I was calling. No call back Monday. I left another message.

No call back Tuesday. (Remember, my patient's surgery was scheduled for that Thursday!)

Then: my scheduler informed me on Wednesday afternoon, the day before the surgery, that the hospital was making my patient sign a document stating that she would pay the bill if insurance didn't, because her doctor did not have prior authorization. Eternally patient person though I am (okay, that's a little humor…), by this time I'd had enough. Picking on me is one thing, picking on my patient is quite another.

I asked my staff to call the patient and her daughter, who was also a patient of mine, tell them what was going on, and ask if they would be willing to call the insurance doctor, keeping in mind that he worked for the insurance company and thus my patient was his customer, not me.

They did call. Then they called me, and told me that the insurance doctor said that I had never left any messages, not contacted him, and had not provided the company with the necessary information to get the surgery approved. Now, I hesitate to use the word "lie," but any other term in this situation would be disingenuous on my part.

So there I was, back on the phone, leaving voicemails as my staff sent her entire chart to the insurance company. (Remember, the biopsy didn't require prior approval; make no sense? I didn't think so.)

Then I called my patient, and while on the phone with her, I got an incoming call from "unknown." I told my patient to hang on just in case this call was about her, though I presumed it was a telemarketer. Turns out it was about her, and it was the insurance doctor.

He said, "Is this Doctor Nomine?"

"Yes."

Then, loudly; "Why did you give my number to a patient?"

I sighed. Then it occurred to me that the patient should hear what was going on, so I merged the calls, and then told the insurance doctor, "You're on a speakerphone."

My patient was smart enough to keep quiet as this guy tore into me, calling me unprofessional and saying it was "callous" to give the patient his phone number.

I said, "What was I supposed to do? I called you Friday and Monday, left voicemails, and you did not call back. Her surgery is tomorrow, and the hospital is making her sign a promise-to-pay for any amounts not authorized because we did not have authorization yet. And what's the big deal, anyway? My patient is your customer, isn't she?

"Yeah, well, I'm going to report you to the insurance company." (Nyah, nyah…)

He continued, "I'll give you the approval for the outpatient work and it will be faxed over in the morning before her surgery."

Then he hung up in my ear.

My patient was quite shocked at how rude her insurance company was to me, her surgeon. She realized it wasn't just the customers who get treated like crap, it was the doctors as well. It seemed a very eye-opening experience for her.

The next day, for a moment, my staff was elated when the fax showed. "Doctor, we got the approval!"

I wasn't ready to pop the champagne cork quite yet. I said, "Let me see that."

I read the fine print and learned that the approval was for an inpatient procedure!

Well, that wily little insurance doctor! He had to know that I had scheduled an outpatient procedure, because that's what we had asked for all along, and on the phone, he had confirmed the procedure outpatient. His actions did double duty, potentially punishing me and the patient at the same time by letting me think we had prior approval, when in fact that approval was for a different location. In this case, the insurance company could deny my patient's claim for lack of prior authorization. Had that happened, neither the client nor I would have a proverbial leg to stand on.

In the end, despite the insurance doctor apparently thinking he could pull a fast one, my staff immediately contacted the insurance company and had them send us a new fax showing approval for outpatient.

Just think of the time wasted by myself and my staff and the added stress my patient had to endure. I was once again reminded about how the insurance companies often get the patient to pay for procedures that should have been covered, quite the same way they maneuver doctors into little or no pay for some of their work.

Making Healthcare More Consumer Friendly

Younger patients increasingly wonder why they can shop for a car online, can order Christmas presents for an entire family within minutes and have them delivered to a dozen different locations, and can plan a vacation over a phone, but they can accomplish nearly nothing to choose their own health care options when they need care.

Health care cost transparency, despite an attempt by the Trump Administration to address it through a 2019 executive order requiring understandable pricing, is highly elusive, as there is rarely an apples-to-apples comparison for surgical services, for instance, that shows a consumer what the true cost is for a hernia operation. Hospitals will either address or ignore this understandable desire by the public. If they're smart, they will take on the challenge. If they're not, prepare for the disruption!

Personnel and workforce will continue to be a challenge for the hospital system, both now and in the future. The young boy or girl from 20 years ago who dreamed of becoming a doctor all their lives may now be disillusioned, frustrated by the system that has cut their pay, increased their hours and left them wondering about their next career. I know that no one cries for the six figure salaries of doctors being shrunk, but it is a fact that excellent students with high technical and scientific aptitude have plenty of other options at this time in history—and the medical profession looks less rewarding than before.

Medical providers must learn how to attract the next generation of doctors and it won't be an easy one. If our country wants the smartest, most capable people going into medicine, then we must pay them accordingly. Otherwise they will go into more lucrative professions like engineering, business, or law.

Finally, how does the health care system function well with reimbursement rates that discourage innovation, new technology, and additional training?

All the symptoms described in this chapter paint a stark picture of a patient in need of some strong medicine, analysis and bold cure. But healing hospitals, health care systems and the myriad of other problems discussed will necessitate leaders from health care, politics, and technology to sit down, grow up, and decide what type of future they want.

Transparency in Pricing

That old saying of "sunlight is the best disinfectant" surely had the health care system in mind, as more health care transparency will make health care better for everyone.

Health care spending has increased nearly 600 percent over the last 45 years, when adjusted for inflation. That means we've gone from spending approximately $1800 per person in 1970 to nearly $11,000 today. (But remember doctor's income per hour worked has been decreasing.)

Pricing competition, of course, like in the case of transparent pricing used by the Surgery Center of Oklahoma mentioned earlier, can provide savings and peace of mind for consumers who feel better knowing the cost.

Dr. G. Keith Smith, M.D. of the Center says, "Hospitals who claim that upfront pricing can't be done, know it can be done. They just don't like what that means for them. They want to work on a 'time and materials' basis, a recipe for waste and inefficiency, as waste and fraud generate more revenue with this model's lack of accountability the more materials used (with their outrageous mark ups) the more they make. Forcing medical facilities to be transparent with legislation is a mistake, I believe, as this is a violation of the quote nonaggression principle quote and also will more than likely provide legislators the opportunity to sell exemptions, with little or no transparency resulting. With the movement for medical price transparency on role now, better, I think, to let the much more unforgiving market deal with those who refuse to be transparent. Those who won't divulge prices will lose out to those who will."

Smith makes a great point on pricing. It may not take a legislative movement to get more transparency in health care. It may just take enough health care systems being shamed by the competitors to get pricing down.

Smith says it may only take a few options to change pricing. "Not all medical facilities need to exhibit transparent pricing in order for a competitive and market economy to emerge in health care. Indeed, our internet pricing has allowed individuals to leverage their local medical facilities, as otherwise they would have gladly jumped on a plane and come to us for surgical care, the price for which was quantifiable. In spite of big hospital's attempts to denigrate this idea, they have found themselves in a competitive environment, whether they like it or not. Whether patients are willing to fly to Costa Rica, New Delhi or Oklahoma City, they have a price in mind in the local hospitals, are shoved against the wall with this pricing, forced to explain why they are 10 times more expensive while simultaneously claiming to not make a profit. In the absence of any evidence that they are 10 times better, their position is a weak one," said Smith. "It's the strangest thing—patients prefer to receive high quality care and not be bankrupted. It sounds radical to say, 'Here's what we do in how much it is.' The mainstream in health care is completely unplugged from the actual cost of the care."

Baylor Scott and White Health, a major Texas health system, has been briefing its patients on cost estimates for major hospital procedures for years. Even walk-ins and ER patients get a good-faith estimate of the price tag. And patients can also use Baylor's online tool that provides an estimate for their specific medical procedures. It's not just a plus for the patients, but it also begins to create additional responsibility on the patient side of the equation. It sets expectations and creates a thought process that allows patients time to decide a) whether they want the procedure, b) whether they should have it at Baylor or shop around and c) hopefully creates an added expectation for full payment by that customer because the sticker shock factor should be reduced.

The upfront pricing has definitely improved Baylor's collections, as it's seen point-of-service payments increase by 60 percent since it started contacting patients with the pricing information! It shouldn't surprise you that treating a customer better and providing them all the information they need provides better outcomes for the health care provider too!

The availability of price information for consumers is increasing. Just about all major health plans offered some sort of cost estimator tool or work with another company to provide one so that patients have an idea of the price. However, many of those tools don't have all of the information necessary to get an accurate price, e.g negotiated rates with providers being included in the calculation, so additional research or phone calls can be necessary.

However, it does make more consumers think through pricing because patients are thinking more about out-of-pocket costs than possibly every before. Why? Surprisingly—or maybe not surprisingly, it's government regulation that has driven up the size of people's deductibles.

One of the byproducts of Obamacare is that many consumers have very high deductibles as part of their health care plan. That means people have more interest in knowing what health care will cost them—or at least, up until they pass their deductible dollar amount. In my opinion, the Obamacare plans are basically a tax disguised as health insurance. For my healthy family of four I paid $2,000 per month with a $15,000 deductible. So basically it was a $24,000 tax I paid to be able to pay the first $15,000 should I need health care. And it was required by law to be purchased. That's extortion. I really don't mind the high deductible plans, but they should cost $100-$500 per month. Not $2,000.

A 2017 study by Health Affairs showed that American consumers with deductibles of $2500 or more were more likely to search for a cost estimate, compare prices or switch doctors than consumers with no deductible or a lower one. What Dr. Smith is saying makes complete sense, as pricing affects other services and products. Look at other industries. When Southwest Airlines enters a new market, fares drop across the board. When Southwest Airlines started flying out of Washington Reagan national airport in 2014, passenger traffic went up 38 percent and fares for all airlines went down 12 percent. Why? To keep their customers from jumping ship, other airlines had to respond and slash their prices to compete!

But that's airlines. How do we get more transparency in health care? We need market forces to work and people to see what a procedure actually costs, but to do that, other steps are necessary. And those aren't as easy because of the giant monster tht is government regulation and bureaucracy. Here's how that plays out in a hospital. Patients have become conditioned to want the immediate gratification of scanners that can detect cancer very quickly. Those scanners cost millions of dollars. Now guess how much of the costs of those scanners can be billed to insurance? Zero!

Why? Because the way the system is designed currently, hospitals and doctors only get paid through patient care services. To buy a PET scanner or CT scanner, health care systems collect money from patients, which pay for the scanners. So whether you get scanned or not, your health care bill includes payments on those multi-million dollar scanners! So price transparency is important, but it's just as important—maybe even more important—to focus on cost transparency. But it's not easy and few people, if anyone, who speak on the subject get it right. When the government agencies overseeing Medicare and Medicaid talk about costs, they are discussing how much consumers will pay in premiums, co-pays, and deductibles. Or, they're talking about how much a hospital says something costs— but every hospital is using different metrics to say what the cost is. Why is this a problem? There's no way to accurately price something when no one can agree on the cost!

Dr. Michael Williams, M.D., director for the Center for Health Policy at the Frank Batten School of Leadership and Public Policy, sums it up best when he says, "No payer—that is, the insurance company for the patient—ever asks about how much it actually costs to provide health care period. Here's why: No one knows. Health care prices are made up numbers."

So what can we do to get a handle on the cost of something? How about we track how much a procedure costs? How much time it takes for procedure to take place? And more: what are the salaries and benefits for the people doing the procedure? What is the purchase price of the machines involved? Does it bother you that none of these things are being calculated right now in most hospitals? If it doesn't, it should!

The Surgery Center of Oklahoma-type organizations know exactly what their costs are. The others are just making guesses. Until we have more accurate cost-determination, we will not get the price transparency we need. And it also won't happen until more of us demand it!

Additionally, keeping doctors in private practice increases competition and lowers the price of health care. If all doctors in an area are employed by a single hospital there is no incentive to keep prices down. Obamacare ruined private practice and encouraged hospitals to "buy" doctors, causing the cost of health care to dramatically increase. This is not due to doctors getting paid more but due to hospitals making more.

Decoding the Billing Puzzle

Have you ever received a medical bill for a surgery, but then another and another comes after it? And another. And you don't even remember meeting some of the people now asking you for money. It's maddening. The people involved are all part of the same system, but it doesn't stop multiple doctors and services from sending you a bill. And in those multiple bills lies potential financial danger because of a sea of billing mistakes that build on each other because of the massive paperwork industry that is the current system. There is always the chance for double billing, inaccurate codes, and the fact that paperwork and payment from the insurance company passes each other in the system and, for example, cause a doctor's bill to show something as 'unpaid' when an insurance check landed in their checking account the same day!

How common are medical billing errors? Very! CNBC looked into billing errors and interviewed employee benefits manager DirectPath. DirectPath found that 50 percent of the bills they reviewed had an error. The American Medical Association lowballs the number, claiming only seven percent of bills contain an error, so assuming the truth is somewhere in the middle of the two numbers tells you that massive billing error rates are shockingly high.

So how can consumers be smarter? Look carefully at your bill and ask for details. Often, the first billing statement a patient receives is a summary with a few generic codes like room charges, laboratory, imaging, and other cryptic entries. That's not what you want—if you get one of the summarized bills and you have questions, call the hospital and ask for the itemized bill with all of the codes included. Once you have that, you are ready to do some detective work.

First, you can start with some deciphering of the codes.

Here are some definitions you need to know.

The HCPCS Level 1, or CPT codes, are five digit codes used by all U.S. medical providers.

The HCPCS Level 2 codes identify products. They usually have a letter in the front of their code (ex: E1234) and are often known as service codes.

ICD-10 codes are attached to a diagnosis. ICD stands for International Classification of Diseases. In the U.S., every service with a CPT code must be linked to an ICD code as a way to make sure the service matches up with the diagnosis. In other words, in theory, they shouldn't be charging for an ankle X-ray to treat a lung cancer patient. If a patient is only being treated for one thing during their appointment or hospital stay, the codes should be the same.

Revenue codes identify the financial amount of the procedure and vary considerably from facility to facility.

So now that you can identify what you are looking at, go online and find a medical dictionary to help you understand what terms mean. If you see things that don't make sense, highlight them and make a note of them.

Then, Google the codes you have been charged for. Google "Medicare code lookup" and you'll find an easy way to find out what a code means. Skip the pricing component of the definitions, as that site is for Medicare pricing. However, finding the definitions through the site is fairly easy.

Also, Google "ICD code reference" and you will find out if you're being billed under the right diagnosis. It shouldn't surprise you that patients have occasionally been billed under the most expensive diagnosis pricing for a service.

So once you have found your definitions, it's time to match up the codes with the charges.

Verify all of the following:

+ Are there double charges? Trust me, it happens. People make mistakes.
+ Did you receive all the services you're being billed for? This includes medications. Know that doctors may order a medication and sometimes it's ignored by someone along the process, but the patient gets charged for it anyway. Watch out for this especially if you were hospitalized. With so many doctors and nurses involved in hospital care, the chance for errors goes up considerably.

- If you were in surgery, think about how long the procedure took and then look at the number of minutes billed for the operating room charge. These times should line up.
- Total everything up and make sure the numbers match the charges.
- If you don't understand something, ask! And ask your insurance company if they have an employee advocacy service for health care claims. If they do, they can be a great resource to help you wade through the maze of codes and mistakes.

All of these steps will help you understand better what you are paying for, but there's one other step to take if something just doesn't feel right. That is, looking into procedure costs and the final bill. While you're out of luck if you're a Medicare patient because costs are what they are, you may be able to use cost look up tools to find out what are reasonable prices in your area for the service you received. FAIR Health (https://www.fairhealthconsumer.org) is a great tool for pricing, but your insurance company portal may have a tool that fits your health care plan also. You can look up some charges by code or service to see if the charges are similar. If you see charges that are higher than normal or unreasonable for your area, you can call to negotiate. It's your right to do so!

Transparency in Outcomes

Patients often here that Dr. Fill-in-the-blank is the best in a certain specialty. And often that is true. But sometimes those comments are driven by the fact that there is a business relationship between the doctor singing the praises and the other doctor.

Wouldn't it be helpful if patients had a better idea of whether the specialist doing a potential life-altering surgery is the best, or if the hospital involved has had positive patient outcomes emerging from it?

Johns Hopkins' Dr. Marty Makary claims, "As many as 25 percent of all patients are harmed by medical mistakes."

In 1989, Dr. Mark Chassin, then-Commissioner of the New York State Department of Health, and his team required all hospitals in the state of New York to report their death rates for coronary artery bypass graft procedures. This procedure was perfect for this experiment because it's highly standardized. "A high death rate is also closely associated with bad judgment, bad skill, and/or recovery care." This information was then made accessible to the public.

After one year, the death rate ranged from one percent to 18 percent. It means some people had one out a 100 chance of dying while others had a one in five chance!

When this news got out, you can imagine the tense meetings and rapid change in hospitals with the high death rates! It caused those hospitals to improve and, over four years, death rates dropped by 41 percent.

It's incredible what sunlight can do. Sometimes, it literally saves lives.

Fixing the System—Stop Making Health Care Harder

Who's CON-ning Who?

Certificate of Need (CON) laws are one of life's many examples of the politicians seeing a problem needing a Band-Aid, but prescribing open heart surgery. CON laws were intended to stop an excess of hospitals from opening in the same area, which assumed that too many hospital beds would mean lots of costs and likely mean increased prices for everyone in the market. What that ignores is that in other parts of the economy, competition works very well, encourages the reining in of costs where possible, and creates efficiencies and expanded choice. But somehow politicians and some health care interests always land on the side of less competition and more rules. It's a protection racket. Competition is good, but unfortunately under CON regulations in many states, competition isn't permitted. Why? The regulations are built in to protect the existing hospitals. CON repeal is one of the few things people from both parties can agree on. The Trump Administration's Department of Health and Human Services supported a repeal of CON, and President Obama did too. Around 15 states have now repealed their CON rules and it's time for more states and the federal government to do the same.

The Best of Intentions—The Worst of Results

During the health care debate spurred by President Obama's election in 2008, people spoke out in frustration about the lifetime caps insurance would place on patients. Insurance companies were portrayed as cruel because a stoppage of insurance payments beyond, for example, $2 million, for someone's health care, no matter how rare, could mean the difference between life and death.

So, caps were legislated into oblivion. But what's happened from there is predictable. Health care tabs for patients have gone up because there is no longer any concern from a hospital about a patient hitting a cap. That's what happens with the combination of the removal of the cap and the "fee for service" model. The "fee for service" is that all-inclusive "buy this IV bag and you're also buying the cost of everything in the hospital" pricing. With no caps, it incentivizes all steps of the health care process to do more procedures, tests and keep patients hospitalized longer. And, insurance companies, while they're paying more to hospitals, charge more to the patients. It's a vicious circle that will not end until "fee for service" is changed and we know the actual cost of a procedure.

Fixing Doctor Flight

Every day, I talk to a colleague who is thinking about leaving the profession. The profession they dreamed about, that they studied long hours for just to have the grades good enough to try to get into a good medical school, and then move onto the fulfilling, well-paying, and honorable job of doctor. It's a shame, but it's not surprising, that many doctors are turning away from medicine and starting completely new careers. But for me, I'm too stubborn and too passionate about the need for great doctors. I'm all in to fight to make our system and our jobs better for this generation of doctors and the ones to come. I'm ready for the fight.

The Association of American Medical Colleges commissioned a 2019 study showing that there will be a shortage of up to 122,000 doctors by 2032. That's a spike from the expectations in the 2017 survey that showed a potential deficit of up to 105,000 physicians.

That's scary and should draw the attention of everyone. We need doctors and our population is continuing to see baby boomers march into retirement in huge numbers, but our system may not have the doctors necessary to treat them. Why?

It's true that some high-performing students that would have been on the medicine track years ago are now looking at a wide array of STEM-related jobs that were not as plentiful, and it's valid to say that some creative minds can become overnight successes without four to eight extra years of college (look at the tech multi-millionaires around the world who haven't turned 25 yet!)

But there's another reality. Being a doctor is not the rewarding job it once was. I wanted to become a doctor so I could change lives for the better in a meaningful way. I gave up some of the years in my 20s when most of my friends were having fun in order to study to reach my dream. And I did. I will never regret that choice.

However, as I talk to my peers, we're often universal in our view that being a doctor today is not the job it once was. It's become paperwork, not people work. Because of arbitrary and constant reductions in payments for medical procedures, specialists are forced to think as much about quantity, not quality, of visits. And huge chunks of our lives are engaged in a constant tug-of-war with insurance companies to simply get paid what we are owed. And with every new page of "health care reform" regulations, our contact with patients shrinks.

And those dynamics are what I believe are causing the shrinking pool of future doctors. The job of doctors has changed—and not for the better. We must fix this now. Imagine what we all thought about family doctors 20-30 years ago if we dropped by with the flu or for a checkup. They sat down with us, knew our names or at least pretended like they did, and had a few minutes to chat about what was ailing us and tell us what we needed to do to feel better.

Today, that same doctor will enter the room, check the charts, ask a few questions and then morph into their federally mandated role of court stenographer.

That shift—and the numerous conversations that take place at doctor's family dinner tables, over coffee, in consultation with aspiring doctors—is driving generational change in people seeking non-medical career options.

This view is shown in research. A 2018 survey by the Harper Poll found that 59 percent of doctors think EHRs (electronic health records) 'need a complete overhaul' and 40 percent see more challenges with EHRs than benefits.

And it's more than just the actions of constantly doing paperwork. At times, the necessity to do paperwork above almost all else can impede health care.

I know of one case where a doctor was treating a child experiencing very serious seizures. The doctor knew instinctively that the child desperately needed medicine in this potentially life-threatening situation but could not legally prescribe the medicine because the child's chart was not yet in the system! That doctor is now a former doctor.

When you get a room of specialists together socially—the ones whose time, talents, and earnings are being squeezed more than any others in the medical profession—you hear as much discussion about what non-medical jobs they are thinking about doing in the future as you do about their current work. It's the open secret and the elephant in the room. And those discussions carry over into discussions with daughters and sons when they talk about careers.

The teenager who watches their mom process billing on Saturdays and Sundays and does paperwork every night is getting a strong, life-shaping message about their next career. Being a doctor means spending most of your time pushing paper. And many of those doctor's kids are listening. We need to change that dynamic now or we'll lose more potential doctors every day.

Curing the Doctor Shortage

I've discussed how some would-be doctors are foregoing the medical profession for business school, STEM careers, or other types of career paths for a number of different reasons, including the quality of the work, the pay, the loss of prestige that comes from spending so much time pushing paper, etc. But complaining is not enough. The health care system needs solutions for addressing the growing doctor shortage. When the U.S. was producing large numbers of doctors, there was a concern that the market would one day be glutted with doctors. As a result, there was a cap placed at 28,000 on how many new doctors could be trained each year. However, that cap is truly unnecessary now, as in 2018, the U.S. produced only 19,000 new medical school students. While it's an increase from 15,500 in 2002, the health care system is falling far short of what we need to keep pace.

One of the big factors causing the shortage has been cost. When a would-be doctor thinks about their future, it's tough to ignore that they will start their careers approximately $200,000 in debt. That's an amount that is tough to pay down even if you're a specialist, but it can be overwhelming for primary care physicians (PCPs), who average a salary of $50-60,000 in their early years. They will eventually make far more, as the average annual pay is close to $190,000 for PCPs, but it's enough of a challenge that it keeps the number of PCPs down. Again, the return on their medical school investment matters. What can be done? There are no easy answers. But we need to find some.

We need more PCPs because, in addition to them being the first step in health care for many people, they're often the most cost effective. PCPs are essential to instilling the importance of preventative medicine, getting the annual checkups conducted, and dealing with many of the factors that are contributing to the expensive chronic conditions that are unnecessarily plaguing so many Americans (diabetes, for instance, costs $327 billion annually—approximately $17,000 per patient with Type 2 diabetes!). If we can cut down on those numbers with proper nutrition and early detection at a lower cost of health care, we can save a lot of lives and billions of dollars. But that means more PCPs!

The NYU Medical School became tuition-free in 2018, but that took a massive fundraising effort that not every school can match. However, in NYUs case, they will produce some doctors who will not be saddled with a mountain of debt. One of the major plusses of NYUs initiative was the massive increase in interest from minority communities. African American applicants jumped by 142 percent that year at NYU! Overall, there was a 102 percent increase in applications from minority students. While some critics of the NYU plan saw a potential watering down of the quality of students if tuition were free, NYU was fast to mention that their standards were not changing—only their tuition was.

NYU's free tuition for medical school was not a taxpayer funded initiative. It came from within the university and they found the donors. While I am not calling for a government funded initiative, there are numerous benefits for finding a way to reduce the cost of or subsidize medical school to help bridge the gap and those solutions could come from the private sector or find creative ways to expand the number of PCPs.

Then there's the National Health Service Corps, a federal program that provides student loan debt relief in exchange for time spent serving in underserved areas. It's a program that can appeal to many medical students, but its budget is currently allowing for approximately 10,000 doctors currently out of the 230,000 in the U.S. When the money is gone, so are the opportunities to participate.

Curing Women Leaving Their Medical Practices

Did you know that almost 40 percent of female doctors either leave medicine completely or become part-time doctors within six years of completing their residencies? That's what the University of Michigan's Intern Health Study showed. Some of the reasons are obvious and likely can't be fixed with a magic wand, but some are not and can be fixed with the right moves.

Family, and specifically having and raising a family, is the biggest reason many female doctors leave. They feel guilt, burnout, exhaustion and think they're not doing any part of their life well. And no matter how equal the genders are in our society, in most households, most women spend a lot more time on parenting and household duties than men...even if the women are doctors. In most careers, women can take some time off if they choose to and hopefully jump back in after a few years. That's not as easy for doctors because of licensing regulations. There is no simple, easy, inexpensive way to take a few years off.

Why, because in most states, all physicians reentering medicine after two years (the length of absence triggering this varies) are required to demonstrate their skills and competency.

And when you take those tests, one of three things can happen.

1. You show that you haven't missed a thing, remember it all and can return to practicing medicine without skipping a beat
2. You show you remember and can do almost everything with skill and proficiency, but will need a period of monitoring to show you are giving high quality care, or
3. You have to repeat some of your residency.

In 49 states, Doctors returning after an absence are required to have some sort of monitoring or evaluation before granting a license back.

Doctors who require monitoring by another doctor for a brief time can expect to pay expensive fees and pay out of pocket for travel and any recommended educational programs to get them up to speed. That is thousands of dollars out of pocket for a doctor who is still paying for their student loans and is currently out of work.

That's expensive for the doctor trying to get back in, but it's also a huge cost for the health care providers who have to go out and hire new doctors to fill those roles. When normal, everyday events like having a child are bringing people to a career breaking point, it's time for creativity that keep doctors in the profession. Thankfully, some systems are starting to provide the thinking that's needed.

For instance, the University of Michigan hospital system has expanded its parental leave policy, which gives mothers 12 weeks paid leave and all new parents six weeks leave with full pay period. Massachusetts General Hospital has launched a parental leave program for all staff in 2018 that gives eight weeks of paid leave for all new parents.

In the University of California Davis Medical Center and the University of Texas Southwestern Medical Center in Dallas have created a "stop the clock" provision that extends promotion and tenure for parents who take leave.

Some systems are considering childcare services and offering of monetary awards to eligible doctors that will provide for dependent care so women can focus on the research and attend conferences and medical society events. These are all creative ways to help doctors manage two very important parts of their lives together and successfully.

What I Love About Medicine

In this book, you've read my profound frustrations with the need for every part of the health care equation—the hospitals, the doctors, the patients, the regulators, and the insurance companies—to improve before we lose the greatness of our system and the values and work that have brought so many wonderful people into the medical profession.

When I think of what I've seen and been a part of, it's been a career and a life that I could have only dreamed of.

A patient review says this: "The doctor found my breast cancer when no one else did! Her expert knowledge helped save my life. I'm very thankful to her."

When I think about those words, I get emotional. While I'd never credit myself for saving someone's life, I was blessed to play a part in making them better and giving them more time with their family. There is no profession that provides the personally rewarding moments quite like being a doctor.

For all the things that bother me about our system, we are in a time of incredible innovation and opportunity. Not all are available today, but breakthroughs may happen in the future on a wide range of diseases and conditions that will change lives for the better and help people in ways previously not thought imaginable.

They include the following:

- Harvard biologist Doug Melton and his team are working on a project to cure diabetes. They are using stem cells to create beat cells that produce insulin. In 2014, he co-founded Semma Therapeutics (named after his two children, Sam and Emma—both diabetics) to develop the project and it was recently bought by Vertex Pharmaceuticals for $950 million. They've created a small machine that holds beta replacement cells, letting glucose and insulin through, but keeping away the problem immune cells. Imagine the lives this one ingenious idea could improve!

- Jonathan Rothberg, a Yale genetics researcher, has created an ultrasound technology on a microchip that can lessen the need for buying a $100,000 ultrasound machine with a $2,000 device that hooks up to an iPhone app. It's not a perfect trade-off with the more expensive model, but it allows for medical imaging to be conducted in poor countries where ultrasounds have always been out of reach.

+ Can you even imagine neurological rehabilitation being sped up by virtual reality—funny glasses and all? Isabel Van de Keere was injured years ago and suffered a spine injury and severe vertigo that forced her into three years of rehab. A Ph.D, she was frustrated by the monotony of the tedious rehabilitation. She's out to change—and speed up—the rehabilitation experience by seeing if VR can help make the process more effective and impactful for attendees and perhaps reduce the amount of time it takes to recover.

+ Peanut allergy therapies have been the dream of many parents for years and hope looks to be within reach. A new oral medicine is being studied that would protect those with the allergy from an attack that can be dangerous for some.

+ 3-D Printing. None of us will ever forget the coronavirus outbreak of 2020, but some innovative people in Italy used 3-D printers to create valves for ventilators after the initial supply ran out. This allowed patients to be treated that likely would not have received all the care they needed.

+ Augmented reality—much like a video game, it provides doctors an experience much like a real surgery that gives them some understanding of what they'll be facing. Imagine a video game with action figures, only in this case it's interacting with a virtual body on the screen. Currently, many doctors performing certain complicated surgeries for the first time get support, but nothing close to the feel of a real-life surgery. AR can provide some of that. For patients as well, it can teach a patient how to apply medication, or rebandage a wound without needing an additional appointment with a doctor. It can reduce errors dramatically, save time, and also save money!

- Vaccine Patches—for those of you who hate getting vaccine shots, one day you might not need them. Researchers have developed a patch with microneedles that inject the vaccine. Eventually, the hope is that it will replace virtually all injects.
- Artificial Intelligence—imagine a computer that can look at pictures of skin cancer and understand what it looks like. According to an article in the *Annals of Oncology*, a computer trained using images of skin cancer has a 95 percent success rate in detecting cancer vs. an 87 percent rate for human doctors.

Engineers at UCLA, UNC School of Medicine and MIT have developed an insulin delivery patch that could monitor and manage glucose levels for diabetics! The adhesive patch could end the unpleasant daily struggle of diabetics, the constant finger pricks and the constant need to adjust to any shift in glucose levels. A game-changer!

And all these innovations, along with the changes and reforms I propose, will save lives and improve our quality of life.

I've told you about the craziness we doctors sometimes encounter, I've described and diagnosed some of the problems, but the reforms and the solutions are what I hope to encourage through my experiences and observations. They mean increased happiness, better lives, and hope for the future—future patients and future doctors.

I'm passionate about making health care better. I hope you'll join me in my mission.

Conclusion:

I love being a doctor, and I especially love being a breast cancer surgeon. The satisfaction I get from seeing women (and a few men) beat the "C Word" and go on to live successful lives with their families makes up for the horror stories I've lived through at the hands of insurance companies.

I love knowing that what I do for a living is perform operations on people who need them—often to survive—not those merely wanting them, often for reasons of vanity other than health. Yes, I could spend much of my professional time performing cosmetic surgeries where cash is paid upfront and no insurance company is involved. But I'd never forgive myself if something went wrong and a patient suffered serious complications from non-essential surgery. I want to be a doctor focusing on the most vital aspect of our profession: saving lives.

Here's something else I want. I want insurance companies to stop interfering in ways that compromise my patients' ability to survive and live healthy lives.

From my point of view, the point of view of the physician, my career and my patient's health care are too often the least of the insurance industry's considerations. Strong words, those, but when big insurance intervenes, when they hire clerks with no medical training and empower them to dictate the course of treatment for my patients, it is the patients who come up short. And this is not mere theory or hyperbole: people's lives are at stake.

I want to take health care decisions out of the hands of business execs and give it back to the doctors and their patients. It seems so simple and logical and self-evident, doesn't it?

Let's make it so!

Additional Reading and Resources

Annals of Oncology
https://www.annalsofoncology.org

Association of American Medical Colleges
https://www.aamc.org

The Journal of the American Medical Association (JAMA)
https://jamanetwork.com/journals/jama

Journal of American Physicians and Surgeons
https://www.jpands.org

Health Care Expense Estimator
https://www.fairhealthconsumer.org

Medical Code Directory
https://www.icd10data.com

Surgery Center of Oklahoma
https://surgerycenterok.com/about/

Ofri, Danielle. What Patients Say, What Doctors Hear.
Boston: Beacon Press, 2018.